T0385433

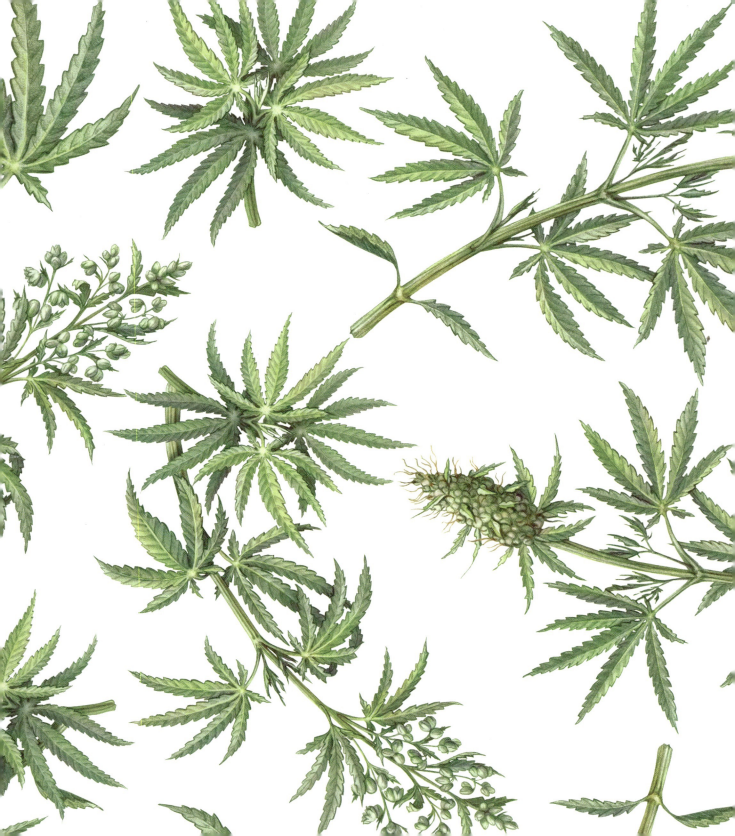

the

CANNABIS

APOTHECARY

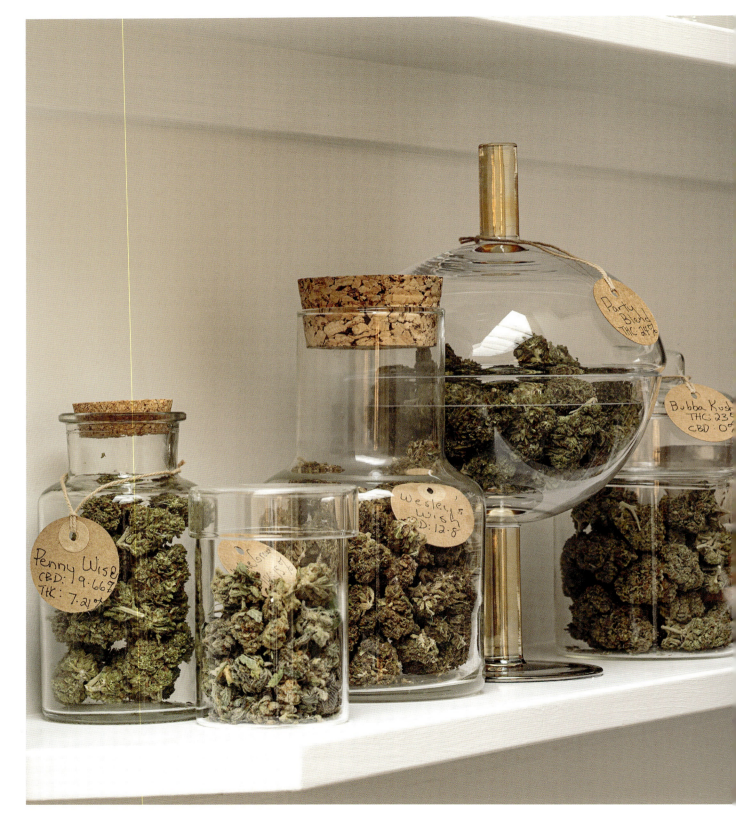

the CANNABIS
APOTHECARY

A PHARM TO TABLE GUIDE FOR USING

CBD & THC

TO PROMOTE HEALTH, WELLNESS, BEAUTY, RESTORATION, AND RELAXATION

LAURIE WOLF

with MARY WOLF

Photographs by Bruce Wolf

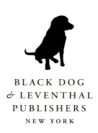

BLACK DOG
& LEVENTHAL
PUBLISHERS
NEW YORK

Black Dog & Leventhal Publishers
Hachette Book Group
1290 Avenue of the Americas
New York, NY 10104

www.hachettebookgroup.com
www.blackdogandleventhal.com

First Edition: November 2020

Black Dog & Leventhal Publishers is an imprint of Perseus Books, LLC, a subsidiary of Hachette Book Group, Inc. The Black Dog & Leventhal Publishers name and logo are trademarks of Hachette Book Group, Inc.

The publisher is not responsible for websites (or their content) that are not owned by the publisher.

The Hachette Speakers Bureau provides a wide range of authors for speaking events. To find out more, go to www.HachetteSpeakersBureau.com or call (866) 376-6591.

Print book interior design by Amanda Richmond.

LCCN: 2019057665

ISBNs: 978-0-7624-9766-9 (paper over board); 978-0-7624-9765-2 (ebook)

Printed in China

1010

10 9 8 7 6 5 4 3 2 1

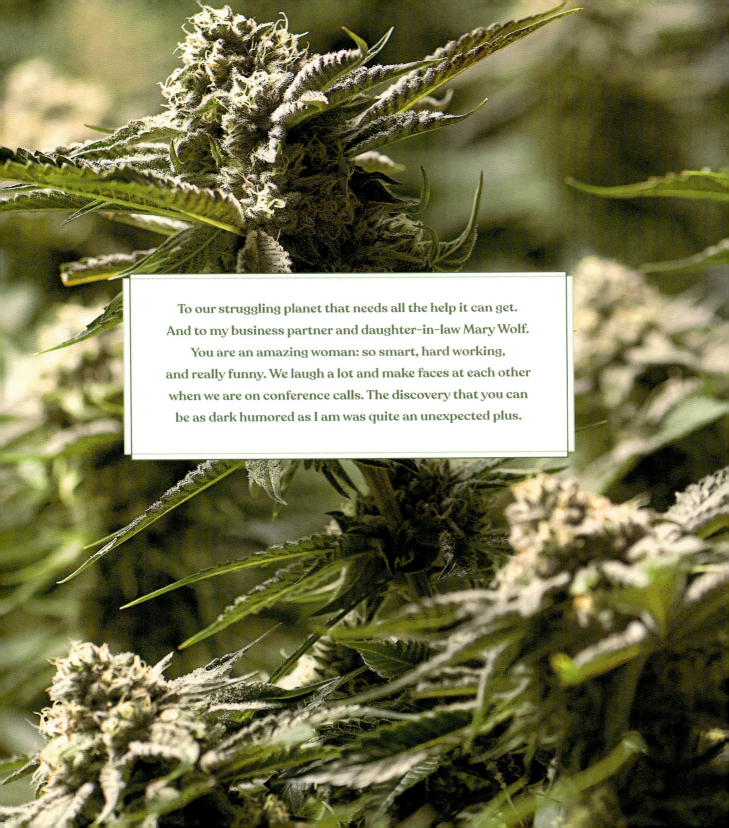

To our struggling planet that needs all the help it can get.
And to my business partner and daughter-in-law Mary Wolf.
You are an amazing woman: so smart, hard working,
and really funny. We laugh a lot and make faces at each other
when we are on conference calls. The discovery that you can
be as dark humored as I am was quite an unexpected plus.

Contents

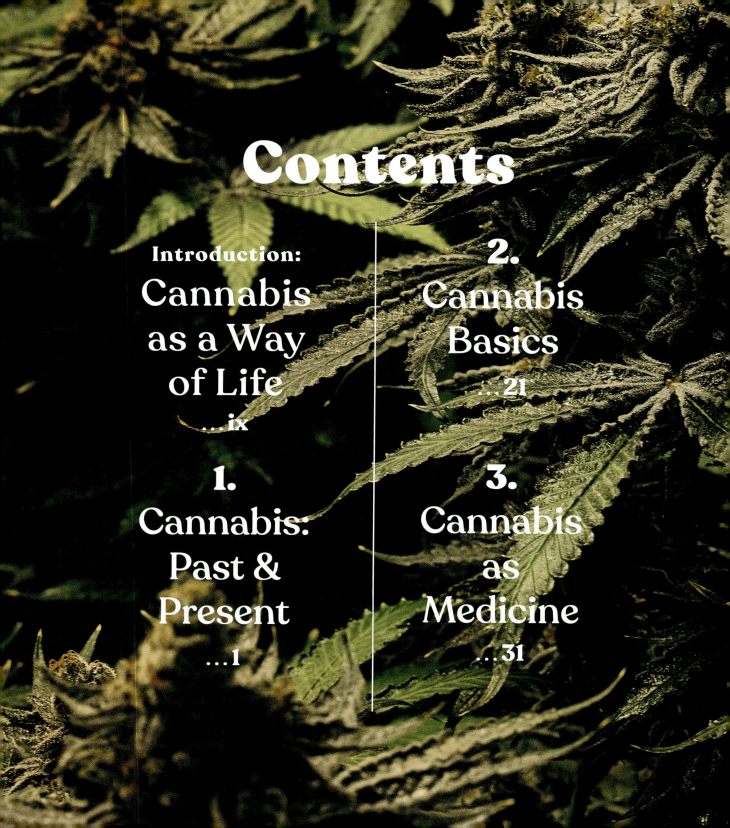

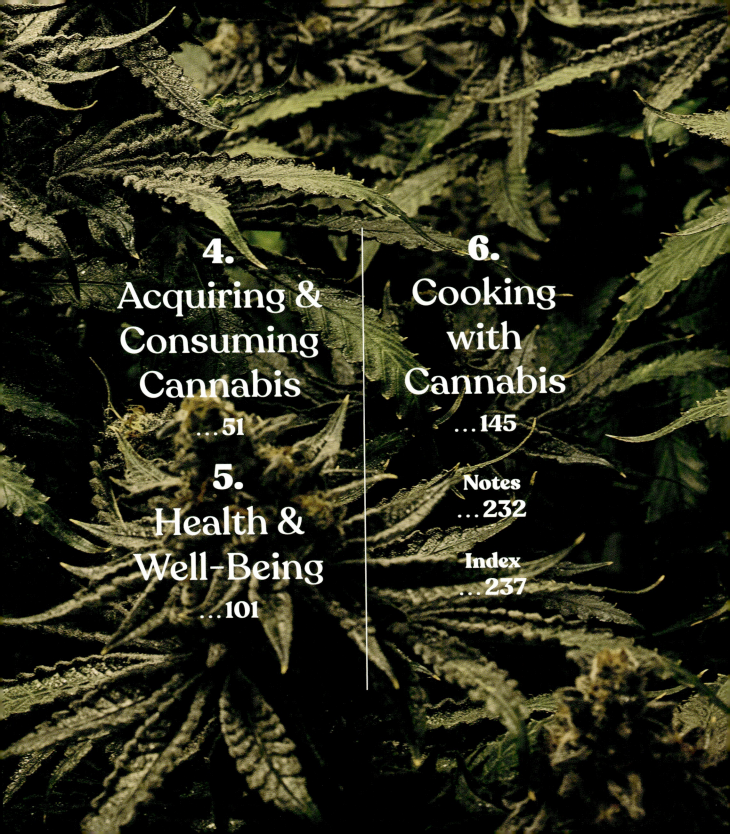

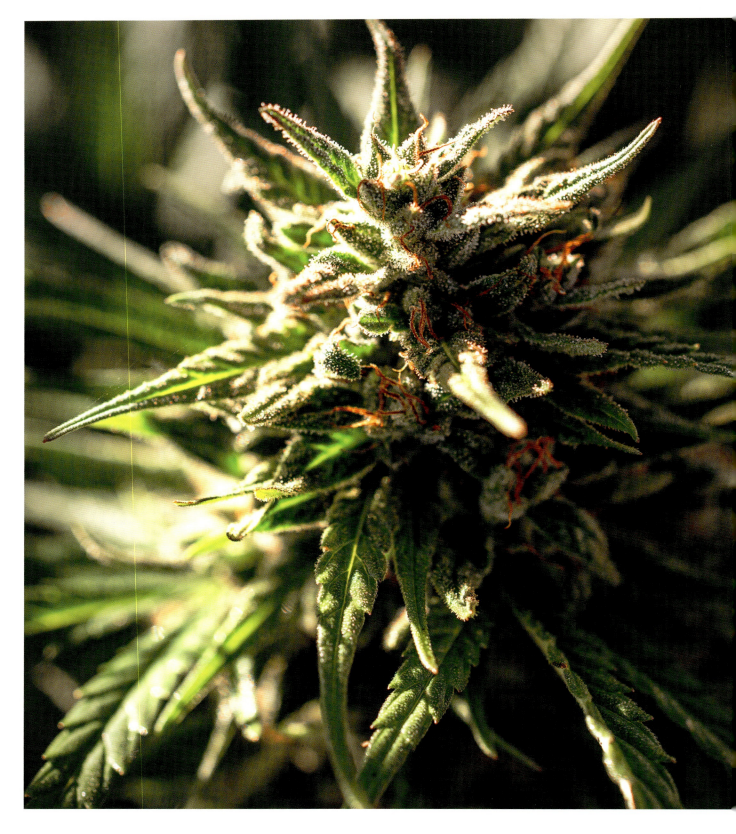

INTRODUCTION
Cannabis as a Way of Life

Almost fifty years ago, my then college-aged brother and I returned to our family apartment to find our mother semi-sobbing. She had attended back-to-school night at my high school and discovered that all but one person in my class was a pot smoker. She said she was hoping that I was that one student, but her tears told a different story. Of course, it didn't help that my brother and I were pretty high while she recounted her story. We tried to tell her not to worry, but we couldn't stop laughing, and I'm not sure how convincingly we made our case. The truth was, we were fine, and so was cannabis. By the end of the evening, we had convinced our mother to try cannabis in an attempt to show her that it wasn't scary or dangerous. She told our dad, and he forbade her to try it. That was back in the day when husbands told their wives what to do and the wives listened.

Wow, how things have changed! Cannabis, both with tetrahydrocannabinol (THC) and without, is part of the lives of many of my friends and, of course, my most esteemed colleagues. Cannabidiol (CBD), now federally legal, is sweeping the nation, and in states with recreational cannabis laws on the books, there has been a huge upswing in cannabis-centered destination tourism. Cannabis lifestyle shops are opening around the country, offering consumers the tools they need to throw cannabis dinner parties and to make their own infused beauty and wellness products. A steady stream of new CBD products is flooding the marketplace, helping people alleviate various aches and pains and improving their sex lives. Cannabis and cannabis by-products have come to play a huge role in the worlds of health, fitness, beauty, and wellness. Even high-end department stores like Barneys are getting in on the action. Their location in Beverly Hills now includes a cannabis lifestyle shop that sells, among other things, a $500 gold-leaf pipe. Cannabis is officially big business, though personally, I prefer an old-fashioned corncob pipe. That's just me.

I am struck by how much of a cannabis lifestyle I have adopted since that night with my mother and brother fifty years ago. What started as the occasional stolen joint as a teen has slowly morphed into a steady daily use of products that positively affect my quality of life. These pot-infused products include edibles, topical ointments and lotions, and pain patches to go along with regular chair massages at my favorite wellness spa in Portland. My hair gets a coconut-infused CBD treatment every two weeks, and my husband microdoses for grumpiness reduction with tremendous results. Even my elderly dogs take CBD for their aging issues!

Cannabis helps me manage both epilepsy and pretty severe depression, allowing me some relief from potent medications that often carry unpleasant side effects, which I'll get into a bit later. My business partner and daughter-in-law, Mary, loves to take a CBD bath and starts each day with our CBD-infused granola. My son, Nick, enjoys a pre-roll when playing video games, including games on a virtual reality console, which is beyond wild when under the influence.

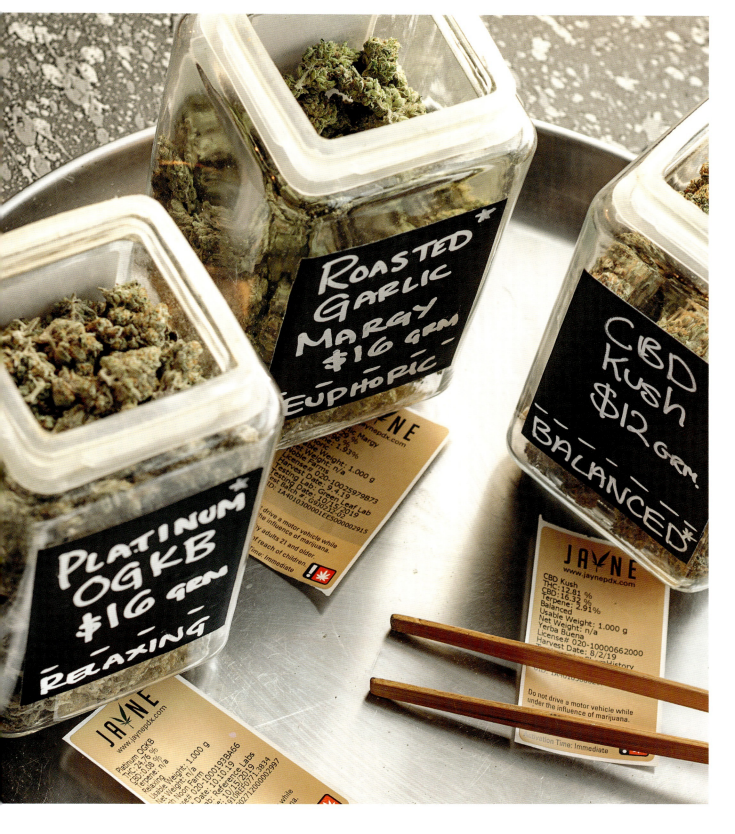

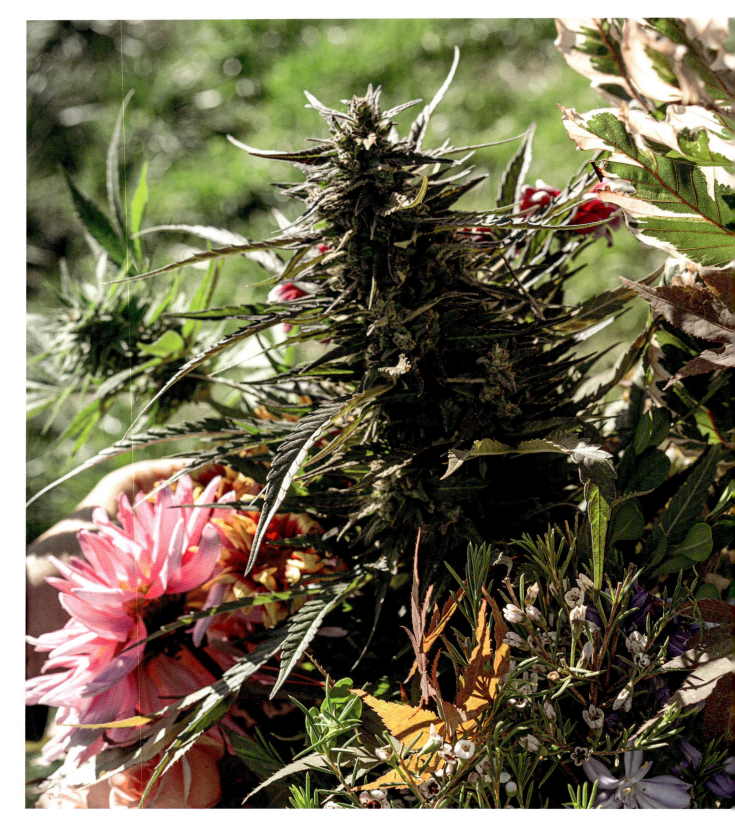

As the nation moves closer to full legality, I've noticed a growing curiosity from people who previously expressed no interest in cannabis. As the stigma surrounding pot recedes, people who once disapproved of the world of marijuana are flooding the market in search of new, interesting, and sometimes life-saving ways to enjoy this spectacular plant. Nowadays there are delivery services that will bring cannabis products right to your door. Here in Portland, a company called Green Box allows you to curate your order online, choosing whatever your cannabis-loving heart desires and delivering your goodies quite possibly on the same day. How's that for progress?

This newfound interest, and the growing service economy that is forming to meet the needs of new consumers, has resulted in exciting new trends in the world of marijuana. Wine-tasting parties are being replaced by cannabis dinners. Older folks with age-related health issues are discovering ways to alleviate their symptoms through pot, and perhaps most promisingly, some studies have shown that marijuana provides a safe, non-habit-forming way for people suffering from opioid addiction to kick the habit.

This book will introduce you to the new and exciting things happening in the world of marijuana. We'll cover all aspects of the cannabis plant, as well as its various recreational and medicinal uses. Whether you're a pro who's looking for fun new ways to enjoy your favorite pastime or a newbie looking for advice on how to manage a chronic health condition in a natural way, we've got you covered. Come and join us as we explore this miraculous plant.

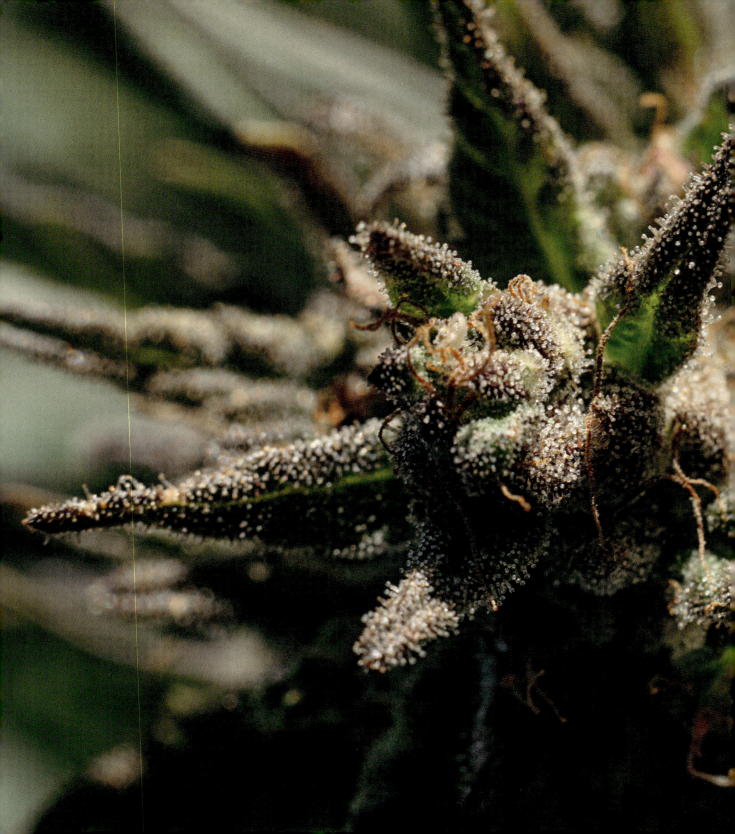

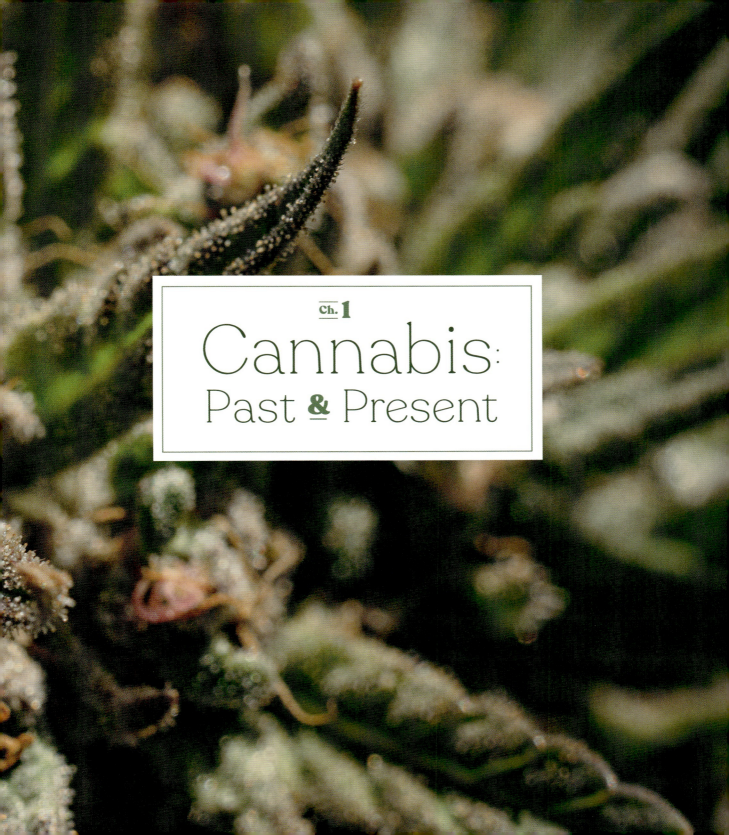

Ch. **1**

Cannabis:
Past & Present

Cannabis has a long and interesting past. The earliest record of the plant comes from roughly twelve thousand years ago. A Neolithic cave painting found in Kyushu, Japan, depicts tall stalks with hemp-shaped leaves featured alongside impressively dressed people, horses, and crashing waves. Dried cannabis seeds have also reportedly been found in excavations of ancient ruins on the tiny island of Okinoshima, off the coast of Kyushu.[1]

More recently, archeologists found proof of the use of the cannabis flower in China's Gobi Desert. Excavations done in the 1990s turned up evidence of an ancient mass burial site from roughly 2,700 years ago. This discovery of two thousand ancient tombs also memorably turned up a large leather basket full of ancient weed.[2] That these ancient peoples were willing to drop a pound of pot into a grave serves as a pretty strong indicator that cannabis must've been plentiful and important in their primitive society, which Dr. David Casarett notes in his book *Stoned: A Doctor's Case for Medical Marijuana*.[3] Tests done by neurologist and cannabis researcher Dr. Ethan Russo and his team revealed that this musty stash contained high levels of cannabinol (CBN),[4] a cannabinoid that is produced over time as THC breaks down. This new information led archeologists to determine that the ancient weed was extremely high in THC. In all likelihood, our ancestors indeed used cannabis for medical and/or spiritual purposes. Cannabis seeds (achenes) have been documented in Chinese medicine for around 1,800 years. To this day, seeds are listed in the Chinese *Pharmacopoeia* for use as a laxative.[5] Cannabis seeds have also been found inside Siberian burial mounds that date back to 3000 BC.[6]

The two men who are given credit for introducing cannabis to the West are Portuguese botanist and physician Garcia da Orta and Irish doctor William Brooke O'Shaughnessy. Da Orta sailed to Goa in the 1530s to serve as the physician to the Portuguese viceroy to the Indies. While in India, he came into contact with the cannabis drink known as bhang. In a book published in 1563, da Orta described his experiences with this strange new elixir: "The Indians get no usefulness from this [bhang], unless it is in the fact that they become ravished by ecstasy, and delivered from all worries and cares, and laugh at the least little thing."[7]

O'Shaughnessy discovered cannabis while in India as well. But in his case, he saw that it was extensively used in medicine, particularly for combating seizures, rheumatism, and spasms caused by tetanus. On his return to England, he published a paper in the *Provincial Medical Journal and Retrospect of the Medical Sciences* attesting to the plant's efficacy for tetanus and "other convulsive diseases," including rabies and cholera.[8] By the late nineteenth century, thanks in part to the work of these doctors, cannabis was part of both the British and American pharmacopoeias.

Medical and Recreational Use in America

Before cannabis was adopted for medical use in the United States, hemp production was actually encouraged by the government. Hemp is a type of cannabis bred for fiber. It does not produce much THC, the main psychoactive element in cannabis. In the seventeenth century, hemp was used as a fiber for rope, sails, and clothing.[9] In the eighteenth century, George Washington famously grew hemp at Mount Vernon and used its fibers to repair the nets he employed on his fleet of fishing boats that trawled along the Potomac.[10]

In the late nineteenth century, cannabis became a popular ingredient in many medicinal products and was openly sold in pharmacies, either in liquid form or as a refined product called hashish.[11] Even back then, the line between medical and recreational use was blurred. A "hasheesh" candy advertised in an 1862 issue of *Vanity Fair*, for example, was billed as a treatment for nervousness and melancholy but was also called a "pleasurable and harmless stimulant." The ad was surprisingly open-minded for its time, encouraging all to partake: "Under its influence all classes seem to gather new inspiration and energy."[12]

The practice of *smoking* cannabis was largely unknown in the United States until it was introduced by Mexican immigrants, who arrived in droves after the Mexican Revolution of 1910.[13] As a result, the recreational use of the drug became associated

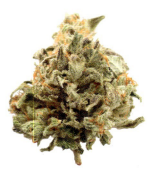

with immigrants even though US citizens had been happily consuming years before their arrival. This incorrect association engendered fear and prejudice not only of cannabis but of the Mexican immigrants themselves. Antidrug campaigners of the day took advantage of the moment and began to campaign against the so-called Marijuana Menace.[14] Between 1914 and 1925, twenty-six states passed laws prohibiting the plant.[15]

By the Great Depression, fear of marijuana was further inflamed by a flurry of research that linked the use of cannabis with violence, crime, and other socially deviant behaviors. By 1931, three more states had outlawed cannabis, bringing the total to twenty-nine.[16] Just five years later, the propaganda film *Reefer Madness* debuted in theaters and further cemented marijuana's poor reputation via a morality tale of "youthful victims" who were lured into trying the drug, only to face terrible consequences.

Prohibition:
Driving Cannabis Underground

In 1937, the US Congress passed the Marijuana Tax Act, which effectively criminalized marijuana by requiring doctors, pharmacists, and dealers to pay a large tax for prescribing or selling the drug.[17] Notably, the American Medical Association opposed the act. This was the start of cannabis prohibition in the United States.

Fewer than ten years later, in 1944, the New York Academy of Medicine issued an extensively researched report declaring that, contrary to earlier research, use of cannabis did not induce violence, insanity, or sex crimes.[18] However, that report was attacked in *The American Journal of Psychiatry*, and throughout the 1950s, stricter sentencing laws were passed, making first-offense cannabis possession punishable by a minimum sentence of two to ten years in jail.[19]

The changing political and cultural climate of the 1960s saw a growing leniency around drug use, including the use of cannabis. Presidents Kennedy and Johnson each commissioned reports that found that marijuana did not induce violence or lead to heavier drug use.[20] Smoking pot seemed harmless and fun, and as journalist Stephen Siff wrote, "In 1967, not only hippie activists but the solidly mainstream voices of *Life*, *Newsweek*, and *Look* magazines questioned why the plant was illegal at all."[21]

Despite the growing cultural acceptance of cannabis, in 1970, President Nixon signed the Controlled Substances Act, which classified the plant as a Schedule I controlled substance.[22] This put cannabis in the same category as heroin—a dangerous substance with no valid medical purpose and a high potential for abuse. Despite the growing call for federal decriminalization, marijuana is still classified as a Schedule I narcotic by the US government. This makes the drug subject to very strict regulations and exceedingly difficult to conduct medical research into the possible medicinal uses of the cannabis plant.

Legalization and Mainstream Consumption

After Nixon's federal cannabis prohibition, several states decriminalized individual possession of the plant, beginning with Oregon in 1972. Other states began to allow for some types of medical and therapeutic use—in 1978, New Mexico passed the Controlled Substances Therapeutic Research Act, which was the first enacted legislation to acknowledge the medicinal value of cannabis. And finally in 1996, California became the first state to legalize the use of cannabis for medical purposes.[23] In 2012, Colorado and Washington state both legalized recreational use, and Colorado became the first state to open dispensaries for recreational use—a novel concept that was quickly replicated by Washington, Oregon, and then Alaska.[24] As of this writing, thirty-three states plus D.C. and Guam have legalized medical use; eleven of those along with D.C. have also legalized recreational adult use.[25]

Medical Uses Today

Despite the lack of large-scale clinical trials in the United States (due to its aforementioned classification as a Schedule I narcotic), cannabis has become an invaluable aid in the treatment of a wide array of diseases and conditions. Published studies from Brazil, Canada, and Israel, countries where cannabis *is* federally legalized, have shown that cannabis is useful in helping to treat everything from autoimmune diseases to neuropathic pain. The drug is approved for treating medical conditions ranging from ALS (amyotrophic lateral sclerosis, or Lou Gehrig's disease) and epilepsy to Crohn's disease, multiple sclerosis, Parkinson's, PTSD, and even opioid dependency.[26] We'll read more about cannabis as medicine in Chapter 3.

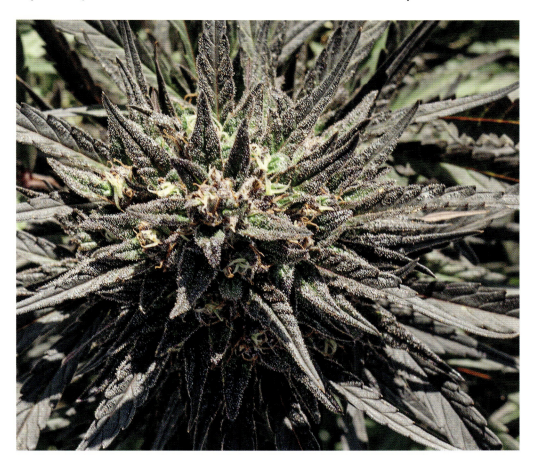

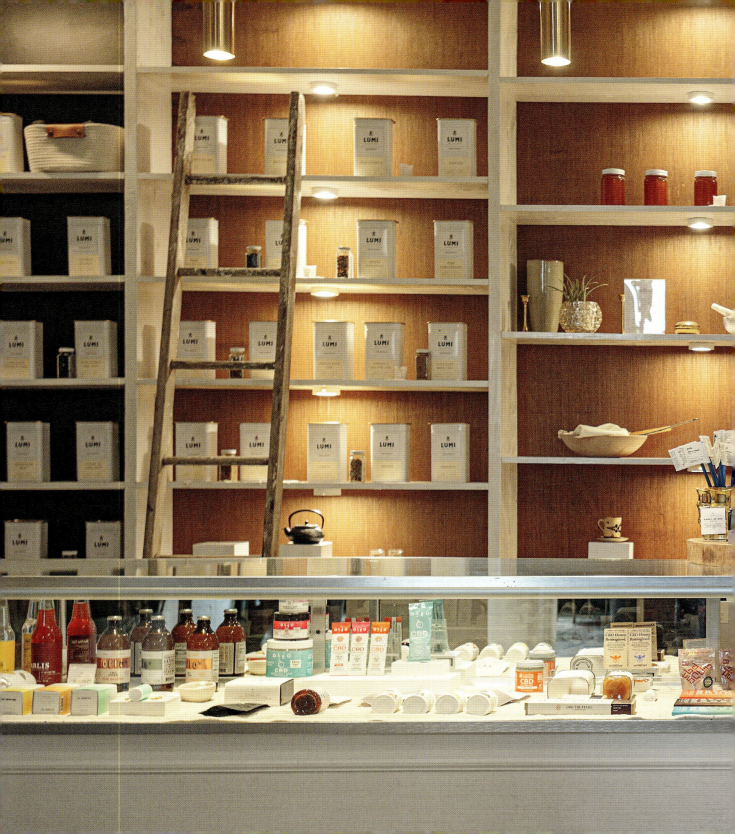

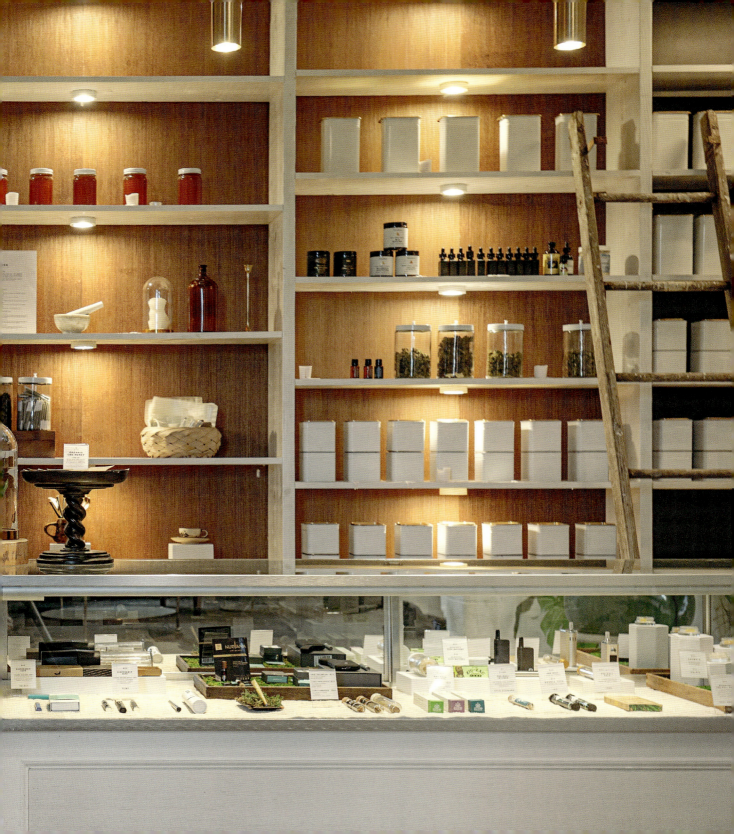

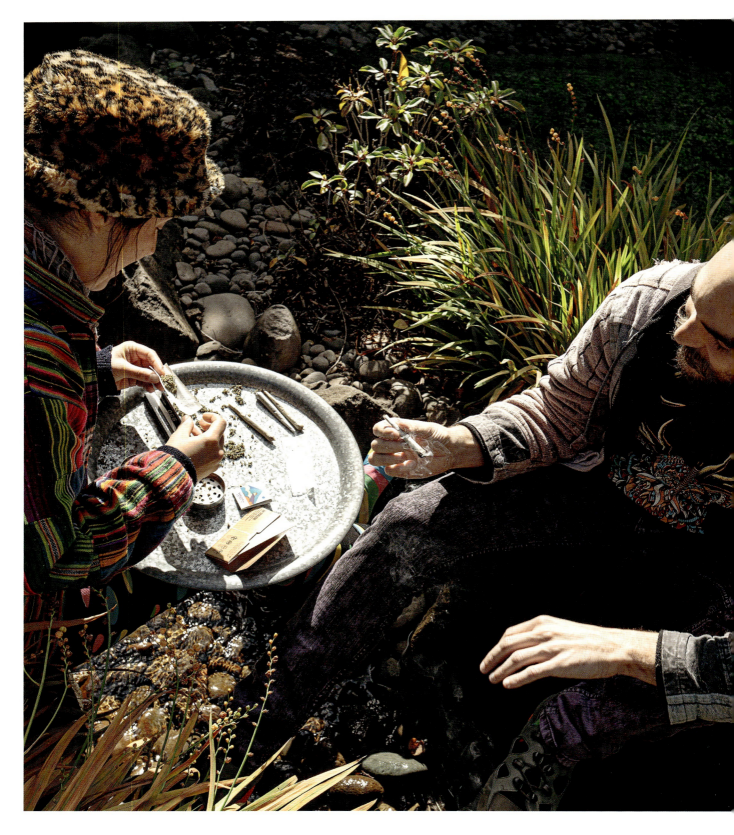

Recreational Uses Today

Cannabis is the third most popular recreational drug in the United States, just behind alcohol and tobacco.[27] According to the latest figures from the *Annals of Internal Medicine*, more than one in seven adults in the US use cannabis.[28] While some of these people are using marijuana for medical purposes, most are recreational users. That means they use cannabis for its psychological and physical effects: relaxation, euphoria, introspection, and even creativity. Today, in states where cannabis is legalized for recreational use, there are yoga and fitness classes as well as spas and beauty studios that promote the careful use of THC and CBD in conjunction with treatments. We'll touch more on this in Chapter 4.

CBD

Cannabidiol, better known as CBD, is a one of a group of chemical compounds found in cannabis. This group of compounds is commonly referred to as cannabinoids. Some cannabinoids, like THC, can have mind-altering effects on your body, but CBD is a nonintoxicating compound that is a potent anti-inflammatory rich in antioxidants. CBD is said to be good for everything from treating blemishes and eczema to helping alleviate anxiety and general pain.

If you're wondering why we've been experiencing a sudden uptick in CBD interest, here's a little background for you. In June 2018, the Food and Drug Administration (FDA) approved a CBD-containing medication, Epidiolex, for use in treating two rare forms of epilepsy: Lennox-Gastaut syndrome and Dravet syndrome. Three months after that, the DEA rescheduled Epidiolex—but not CBD itself—to Schedule V, which means it has an accepted medical use and a low potential for abuse.[29]

Other than the drug trials that were administered in order to get Epidiolex approved, most of the published research on CBD comes from preclinical studies, which are often done on animals or in a petri dish, not on humans. The standard double-blind, placebo-controlled human studies that the Western medical establishment favors are only now being run, after the FDA relaxed restrictions in December 2015.

We still have so much to learn about the efficacy and uses of CBD, but that hasn't kept it from becoming ubiquitous as the wellness ingredient du jour. CBD can be found in everything from mascara to cocktails. A grocery store in Oregon even sells a CBD-infused bratwurst! According to the Chicago-based Brightfield Group, sales of CBD-based supplements, personal care products, and food grew by 88 percent between 2016 and 2017, earning a total profit of $327.4 million. With the legalization of hemp under the 2018 Farm Bill, the CBD market was projected to skyrocket to $5.7 billion by the end of 2019.

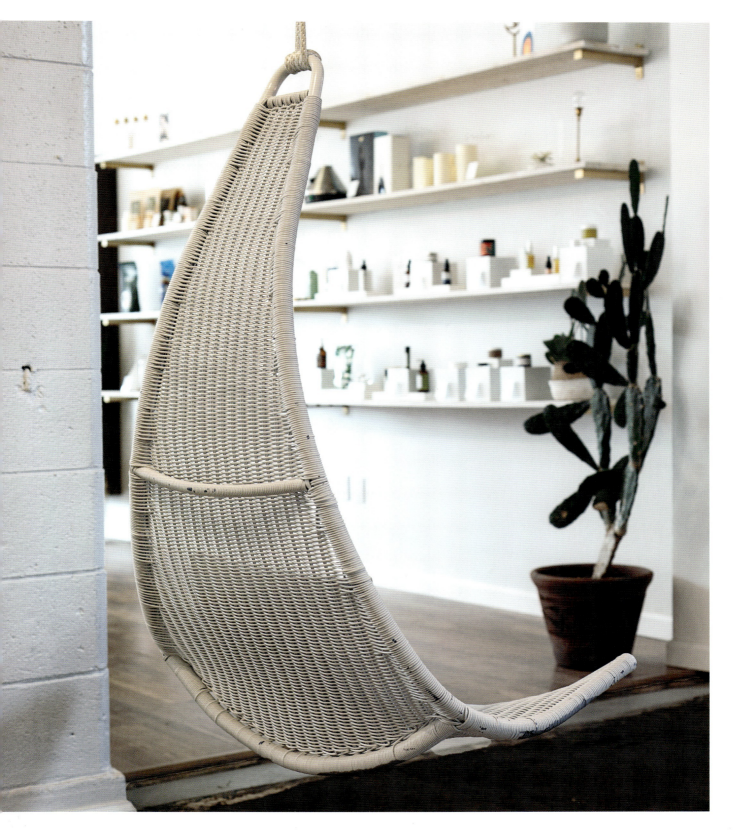

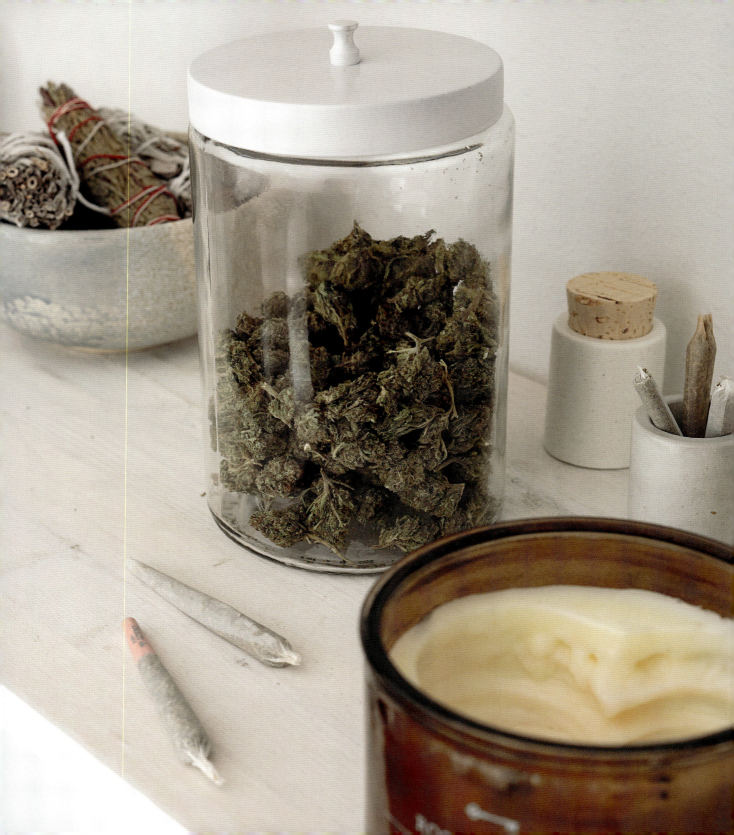

As mentioned earlier, hemp is a variety of cannabis that has traditionally been used to make clothing, rope, textiles, and paper. It has specifically been bred over centuries, possibly millennia, to contain as little THC as possible. In the US, hemp is legal as long as it contains only 0.3 percent or less of THC. Until recently, CBD was also legal only if it came from a state that grew industrial hemp under the provisions of the 2014 Farm Bill. But when Congress passed the 2018 Farm Bill, hemp—and therefore CBD— was declassified at the federal level, making it easier to grow and to ship across state lines. Under the new law, which took effect on January 1, 2019, hemp plants containing no more than 0.3 percent THC are no longer classified as a Schedule I controlled substance. "This is nothing short of seismic for the cannabis industry," said Kristen Nichols, editor of *Hemp Industry Daily*, in an interview with *Bloomberg*.[30]

This means that farms all across the country can—and are—growing hemp legally. Some craft cannabis farmers, like brothers Aaron and Nathan Howard at East Fork Cultivars in southern Oregon, are breeding new strains of hemp that contain even higher levels of CBD. Traditionally, hemp has had low resin, and so contains only small amounts of CBD—not a medicinally important amount. The Howards also sell plants on their recreational cannabis site that are higher in CBD than most THC-containing strains have been in recent decades. CBD, in addition to its many other benefits, can ameliorate some of the negative side effects of THC.

Anna Symonds, director of education at East Fork Cultivars, teaches a free CBD Certified class for frontline cannabis professionals in which she details the latest research about CBD and how it works in the body. Preclinical research has shown that CBD is analgesic, antianxiety, antiseizure, neuroprotective, anti-inflammatory, antitumor, and even antipsychotic.[31] It can also help lift mood and depression, probably because it interacts with serotonin receptors. In addition to being nonintoxicating, CBD is also nontoxic and nonaddictive—even at high doses. According to Symonds, the only side effects of CBD are positive: It can lower blood pressure and reduce a type 2 diabetic's need for insulin (though she counsels people to take CBD at a different time of day than they take other medications, just to discourage potential drug interactions.)[32]

Like THC, CBD interacts with your body's endocannabinoid system (ECS). The ECS, which was only discovered in the 1980s,[33] has receptors all around the body. CB1 receptors are found mostly in the central nervous system (brain, spinal column, and nerves), and CB2 receptors are found mostly in immune system cells and in the gut. Interestingly, scientists have found that CBD activates CB1 receptors only when THC is present. This is probably why small amounts of THC used in conjunction with CBD are better for remedying analgesic and anti-inflammatory conditions. For this reason, Symonds and other cannabis educators refer to CBD and THC as "the power couple." CBD doesn't bind directly with CB2 receptors, but there is speculation that there's some kind of indirect action that helps. We'll read about the endocannabinoid system in more detail in Chapter 2.

Q & A
WITH ANNA SYMONDS

Talking to Anna Symonds, director of education at East Fork Cultivars, a leading craft hemp and CBD-rich cannabis farm in southern Oregon.

Symonds, thirty-eight, has taught East Fork Cultivars' science-packed CBD Certified class to budtenders, growers, and producers for two years. Over that time, she has crisscrossed Oregon, teaching the class at over one hundred dispensaries and industry conferences. "It's always free," Symonds says. "It's a very mission-driven program. We want people to have information—to be empowered to take care of their health." Recently, she launched CBD Certified Live, an online version of the classes, which allows people from around the country and world to learn about CBD. We asked Symonds to share her passion for CBD—and a few basic tips on how to enjoy its benefits.

☘ How did you get interested in CBD?

I'm an athlete. I play rugby—a contact sport—and it's pretty intense. I heard about CBD in 2014 from a friend in the Bay Area. I started reading what I could and tried to seek it out, but it was still more rare to find CBD-rich cannabis. When you did, it was often sketchy or it had just a little bit of CBD—and you never knew if the same thing would come back. I didn't reliably start a regimen until about 2016. It's made a big difference to me.

☘ What's your favorite way to use CBD?

As a supplement, I find capsules very convenient and tinctures versatile. For immediate pain relief and muscle relaxation, I prefer to smoke cannabis—with varying ratios of CBD and THC. It's the best consumption method for me. Topicals are great for people, but they're not as systemic—they're localized, as the skin is still a barrier. I generally need anti-inflammatory effects throughout my whole body, and when you get it from within, the anti-inflammatory action is more powerful. But I definitely do use topicals for some extra help in painful spots or in bath soaks. And, of course, there are some delicious foods and treats infused with CBD as well.

🌿 In your Certified CBD class, you emphasize that in most cases a tiny bit of THC will help potentiate the CBD. Why is that?

THC is a more potent analgesic for acute pain than CBD is. (Though CBD is a potent anti-inflammatory.) If I need pain relief, I'm definitely going to go toward higher THC content—though still with some CBD in it, too. I know that that works for me. And it's not just for pain relief—I'm stopping muscle spasms. Relaxing my muscles that can get incredibly tight and painful. I've found cannabis to be the best muscle relaxer.

The research on sleep is interesting: THC helps you go to sleep faster, but CBD promotes more quality sleep.

🌿 How did you become a CBD educator?

It's by chance that I even got into the cannabis industry. I did some consulting for a grower. Through that, I learned more about the industry and got immersed in everything cannabis: land use, cultivation, OSHA, finances. And East Fork Cultivars [which is known for its focus on high CBD strains] was a company I really admired. I was lucky enough that the East Fork partners wanted me to build and run their education program. It helped that I had an academic background in communication and a passion for CBD.

🌿 With CBD lining grocery store shelves in most states, how do consumers ensure they're getting the best-quality CBD?

It takes some work. We're coming out of Prohibition—we don't have the infrastructure yet. It can't be USDA certified organic unless it's hemp (which, by law, must contain less than 0.3 percent THC). So if you can't get that, look for US grown and ideally organic. There are three certifications for organic cannabis: Clean Green, Dragonfly Earth Medicine, or Dr. Bronner's new Sun+Earth.

Full-spectrum products—not made of CBD isolate or distillate—will offer the greatest range of potential therapeutic effects and a greater value for your money. Make sure that the product offers test results from a third-party accredited lab. Avoid additives like artificial colorings and flavorings, "food grade" terpenes, sugar, and preservatives. Be very careful and skeptical of vape cartridge additives. You should not be inhaling things like MCT oil or other thinning agents, essential oils, or other flavorings.

There are a lot of people who are selling inferior products. Vote with your dollar— buy from companies that will not only provide you with a safe and effective product but will also support your personal values.

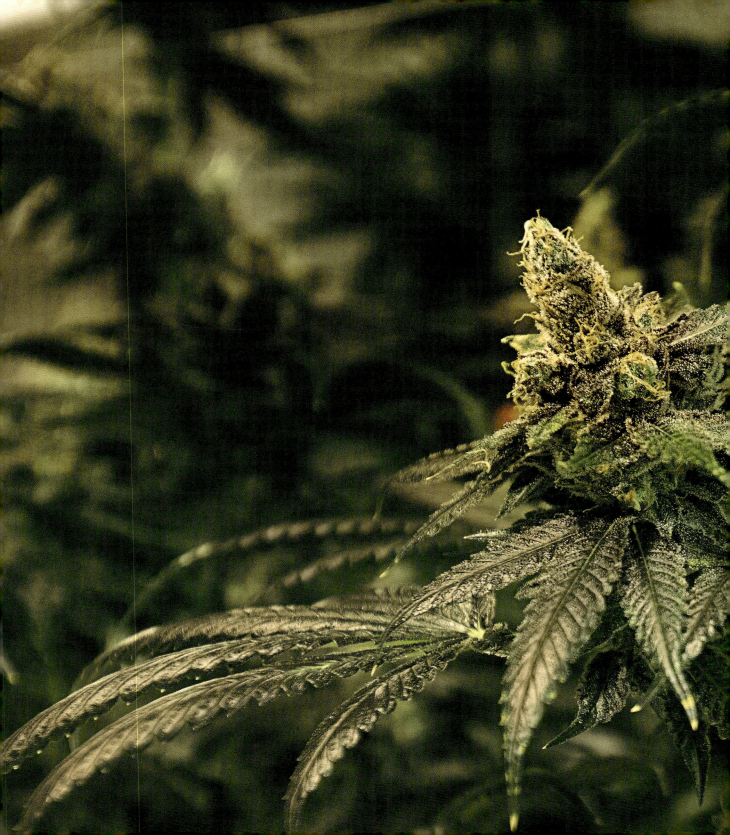

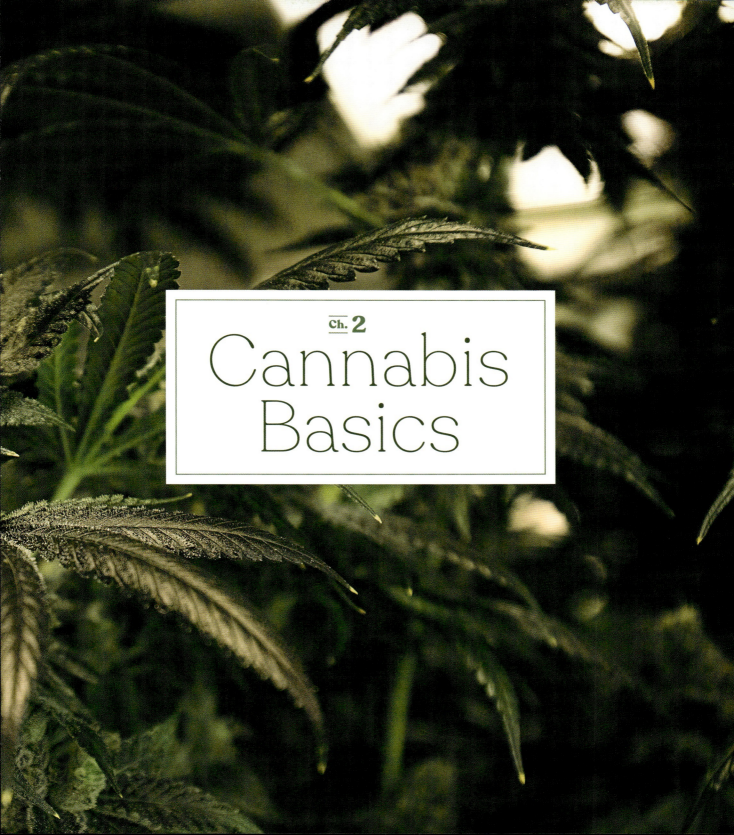

Ch. **2**

Cannabis Basics

Whether it is smoked, infused into food, or applied topically, the effects of taking *Cannabis sativa* can vary in ways that are sometimes hard to explain. But I will try my best, with a little help from my friends. The lovely cannabis plant can be used to treat quite a range of issues, from helping to reduce anxiety, inflammation, and pain to promoting appetite, cell regeneration, and immune support. How can one plant do all of this? you (and I) might wonder. To answer this question, we need to step into some science.

The Endocannabinoid System

The chemical compound THC was officially named and labeled in the 1960s by scientists who were studying the effects of cannabis on humans. Over the years, researchers worked to understand how, exactly, THC affected the body, and this led them to discover a network of receptors within the body that sparks a reaction when it comes into contact with THC. These receptors make up what scientists now refer to as the endocannabinoid system, and they are responsible for regulating the homeostasis (balance) of all of our most basic biological functions.

Endocannabinoid receptors are found in the brain, internal organs, central and peripheral nervous systems, cardiovascular system, reproductive system, gastrointestinal system, urinary system, immune system, and even cartilage. They are everywhere in your body, which helps explain how and why cannabis is used to treat so many conditions. The endocannabinoid system helps regulate appetite, metabolism, sleep, memory, female reproduction, immune response, and pain. Since its discovery in the 1980s, the endocannabinoid system has been appropriately considered the most important system in the human body.

Shortly after the discovery of the endocannabinoid system, researchers defined two varieties of receptors within the system: CB1 and CB2 receptors. Found predominantly in the central nervous system, CB1 receptors are the most prevalent receptor type in the brain and spinal cord, and they are responsible for producing the "high," mind-altering effects of cannabis. CB1 receptors have also been linked to regulation of memory, motor skills, appetite, pain, mood, and sleep and are thought to aid in neuroprotection[1] and neurogenesis[2] (good news for potential treatment of Alzheimer's, Parkinson's, dementia, and multiple sclerosis). CB2 receptors are found predominantly in the immune and peripheral nervous systems, and they do not produce psychoactive effects. When activated, CB2 receptors promote anti-inflammation and pain relief. Though they are typically found in different areas of the body, both CB1 and CB2 receptors can occasionally be found in the same tissues, but when activated, they produce very different effects.

Now for something pretty cool: Because the endocannabinoid system is all about regulating our internal homeostasis, a couple of interesting things happen when you consume external cannabinoids, or phytocannabinoids (i.e., marijuana). Researchers found that the introduction of cannabinoids stimulated the creation of more receptors in the endocannabinoid system, thereby increasing a person's sensitivity to the cannabinoids they consume after this initial introduction. This may explain why sometimes people experience cannabis more acutely after their first try. However, if you overdo it and start intaking too many cannabinoids, the endocannabinoid system may start to reduce the amount of receptors, decreasing your sensitivity and increasing your tolerance. So if you start to feel as though you need more cannabis than you used to consume in order to achieve the same effects, take a month off and see what happens when you return. A month of abstaining may reset your system and your tolerance.

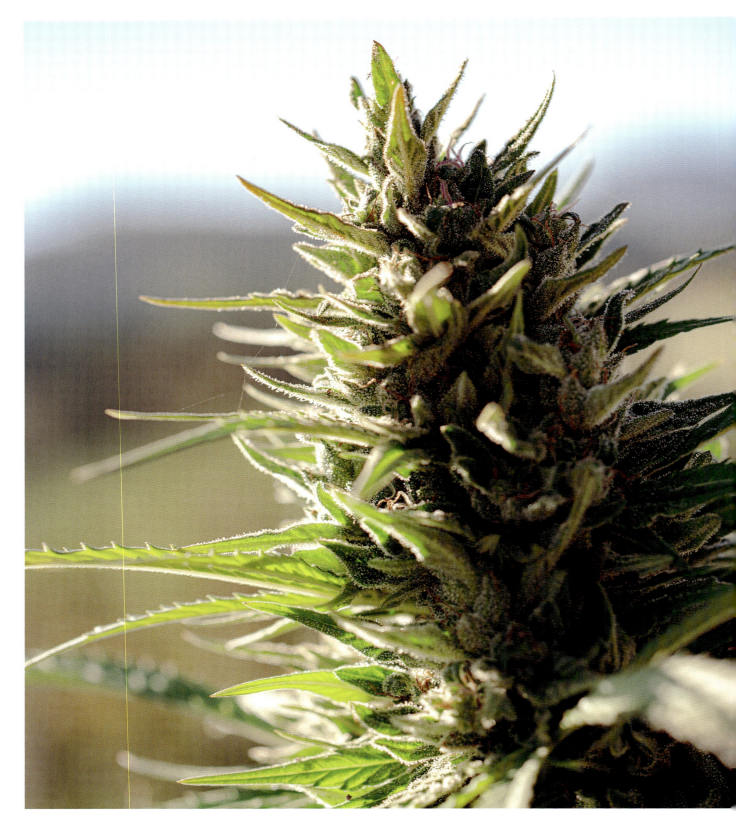

Cannabinoids: THC & CBD

Our bodies naturally produce chemicals called cannabinoids, which activate and regulate the endocannabinoid system. Cannabinoids are also found in the cannabis plant and are referred to as phytocannabinoids—so named because they are plant-based. These phytocannabinoids are found in the plant's resin, which concentrates most heavily in the buds of the plant.

THC (short for delta-9-tetrahydrocannabinol) is the most famous (and infamous) of the phytocannabinoids; it is also the most abundant and is responsible for the psychoactive effects of cannabis as well as for many of its medical benefits. THC mimics naturally occurring cannabinoids already present in the body, which are responsible for thinking, concentration, perception of time, pain, and pleasure. THC activates CB1 and CB2 receptors and helps to reduce pain and promote anti-inflammation as well as to stimulate the appetite and reduce nausea. It also appears to protect the brain and stimulate neurogenesis.

Raw cannabis actually produces tetrahydrocannabinolic acid (THCA), which, once heated, becomes THC. THCA is not psychoactive, but it does have its own medicinal benefits, such as anti-proliferation, anti-inflammation, and neuroprotection. Eating raw cannabis would not get you high. Heating cannabis releases carbon, through a process called decarboxylation, which converts THCA into THC.

At this point we might as well mention THCV, or tetrahydrocannabivarin. This cannabinoid is similar in structure to THC but produces its own specific effects, like appetite suppression, diabetes support, anxiety reduction, Alzheimer's support, and bone growth. Like THC, THCV is psychoactive and has been said to produce euphoric highs that are stronger and faster than the effects of THC alone.

Growing in popularity and interest is the second most abundant cannabinoid found in cannabis, CBD, or cannabidiol. It activates receptors in the CB2 receptor system and as such is not psychoactive. Like THC, CBD has also been shown to produce pain relief, anti-inflammation, anti-nausea, and antianxiety. CBD is also anticonvulsive and can be used to treat epilepsy. In fact, research suggests that patients found greater relief from using a combination of CBD and THC than from using either cannabinoid on its own. As with THC and THCA, CBD begins its life as cannabidiolic acid (CBDA) before it is decarboxylated by heating. Research has reported therapeutic benefits of CBDA, such as treating side effects of cancer like nausea, as well as inflammation.[3]

Although THC and CBD are the most well-known and abundant cannabinoids, the list goes on, including CBG, CBN, CBDV, and CBC, all of which are not psychoactive. Cannabigerol (CBG) is like the mother cannabinoid—it is the precursor from which all other cannabinoids are derived. CBG interacts with CB1 and CB2 receptors but can act as an inhibitor to the psychoactive properties of THC. It has also been shown to be anxiety reducing and to help relax aching muscles. Plants that are harvested early usually contain traces of CBG. And on the flip side, THC and CBD both degrade into CBN. CBN may help fight bacteria and act as a neuroprotectant and anti-inflammatory. It is also relaxing and reported to be very sedating. CBC is also produced by CBG. It works within the endocannabinoid system to promote production of natural endocannabinoids within the body. CBC has demonstrated anticancer and antitumor properties and offers promising therapeutic benefits.

Terpenes

Research into cannabis has mainly focused on the plant's cannabinoids, but terpenes are the next frontier. Like cannabinoids, terpenes are located in the plant's resin. They give different marijuana strains their distinct smells, tastes, and (to a certain extent) effects. Terpenes are also found in other plants, including fruits, herbs, spices, and flowers. We consume terpenes every day, in foods like mangoes and lemons, and spices like black pepper and bay leaves. Terpenes have a wide range of physiological manifestations that closely mirror the prized medicinal uses of cannabis. They can be used to ease anxiety and inflammation, general pain, epileptic seizures, and more. Each terpene contributes its own set of attributes, which work in tandem with a plant's cannabinoids to produce the overall bodily effect of an individual strain of marijuana. This combined effect is known as the "entourage effect." Researchers have found that the full spectrum of healing properties found in cannabinoids and terpenes are strongest and most beneficial when used in their naturally occurring states, rather than using a distilled and isolated cannabinoid or terpene on its own.

MYRCENE

The most predominant terpene in cannabis, myrcene has properties that are sedating, muscle-relaxing, painkilling, and anti-inflammatory. Myrcene is also found in mangoes, hops, lemongrass, thyme, and sweet basil.

LIMONENE

Found in citrus peels, rosemary, juniper, and peppermint, limonene can promote weight loss, elevate your mood, and relieve stress. It fights inflammation, pain, and even cancer.[4]

LINALOOL

Found in lavender and mint, linalool is often used in cosmetic products because of its natural floral fragrance. It is both sedating and pain-relieving and can act as an antianxiety, antipsychotic, and antidepressant aid.

CARYOPHYLLENE

This terpene has a rich fragrance that is equal parts spicy, peppery, and woody. It is antiseptic, antibacterial, antifungal, and anti-inflammatory—good for arthritis and autoimmune disorders. Caryophyllene is found in black pepper, cloves, Thai basil, and cotton. Research suggests it interacts with CB2 receptors in a way that mimics CBD.

PINENE

The terpene that gives many strains their sweet, piney scent, pinene promotes alertness, memory retention, and anti-inflammation and helps to relieve asthma. It may also counteract the psychoactive effects of THC.

TERPINOLENE

Terpinolene is one of the least common terpenes in cannabis. But with anticarcinogenic, antioxidant, antifungal, antibacterial, and anti-insomnia benefits, this terpene is not insignificant. Found in apples, cumin, tea tree oil, and lilacs, its fragrance is often described as woodsy and smoky.

Cannabis vs. Hemp

Would it surprise you to know that the distinction between hemp and cannabis is purely a legal one? It sure surprised me! Cannabis plants that contain 0.3 percent or less of THC (by weight) are classified as hemp. It is that simple . . . and confusing. It all comes down to the THC content. For me, "cannabis" means THC and "hemp" means CBD. I know both can have other cannabinoids, but essentially, in my view, when you're going for cannabis, you're going for the THC (or a ratio incorporating THC), and when you're going for hemp, you are hoping for some natural CBD. Did you know that the hemp plant was brought to the US on the *Mayflower*? And, as we previously mentioned, that George Washington grew (and smoked) hemp? Of course, back then there weren't labs to test the THC content, so who knows.

The More You Know:

If you see "hemp seed oil" or "cannabis sativa oil" listed in the ingredients of commercially available products, this does not necessarily mean that these products contain THC or CBD. If you don't see specific amounts of THC and CBD listed, chances are there aren't any. Hemp seed oil and cannabis sativa oil are made simply by pressing the seeds of cannabis and hemp plants. They may come with their own set of benefits, but they should not be confused with oils from the cannabis flower itself.

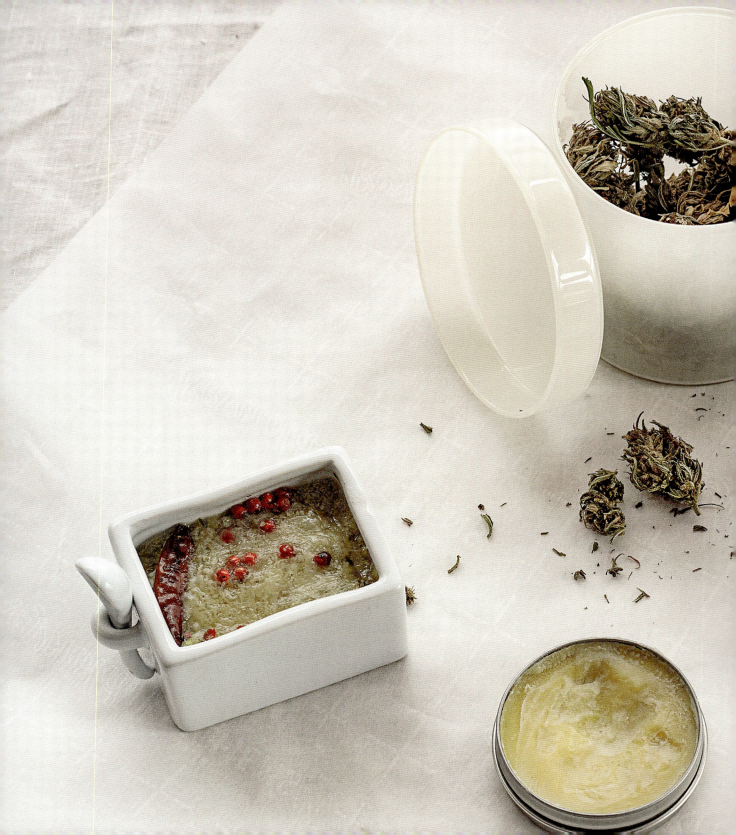

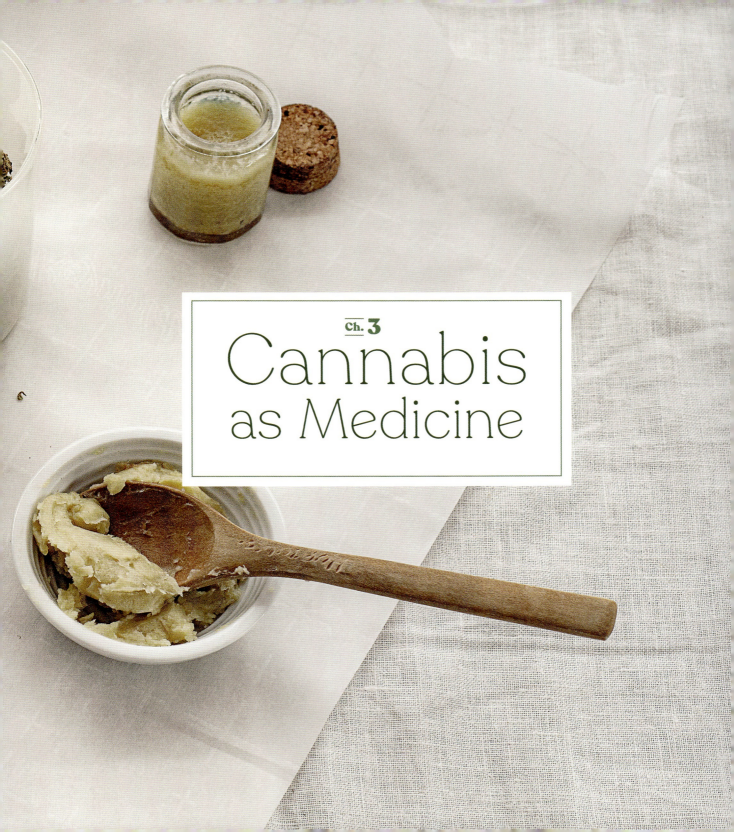

Ch. 3

Cannabis as Medicine

One of the world's oldest medicines, cannabis has endured for centuries (possibly millennia) as a treatment for a wide variety of ailments. Cannabis research continues to find promising medicinal applications for this lovely herb, which can be used for everything from pain relief and anti-inflammation to treatment of insomnia and epilepsy. I, for one, have used cannabis medicinally for the past six years to manage my own epilepsy.

THC may be the best-known cannabinoid, but it alone is not responsible for all of cannabis's beneficial effects. As discussed in Chapter 2, research suggests that cannabinoids and terpenes, as well as other chemical compounds, all work together to help deliver what is known as an entourage effect.[1] That's why taking full-spectrum sources of cannabis or hemp (that is, sources that have not been distilled or isolated) are more effective than taking diluted forms of marijuana.

For a long time, research into cannabis was essentially limited to its potential negative effects: Is it addictive? Is it harmful? Needless to say, if researchers or government agencies found any solid evidence to support either of these questions, we'd all be *well* aware. As legalization efforts progress, research into the health benefits of weed has expanded and grown. Scientists are now looking into potential marijuana-based treatments for Alzheimer's, cancer, Crohn's disease, and ALS. While more studies are needed to explore the full range of possible treatments, evidence has already been found that supports the use of marijuana to help alleviate or treat the following conditions.

Pain

Cannabis is widely used to relieve pain, especially chronic pain. In fact, pain management is one of the most commonly reported reasons patients give for using cannabis. A 2013 review published in *The Clinical Journal of Pain* found thirty-eight randomized controlled trials (the gold standard for medical research) that studied the relationship between cannabinoids and pain management. Twenty-seven of these trials showed that cannabinoids had "demonstrable and statistically significant pain-relieving effects."[2] Even more recently, in 2017, the National Academies of Sciences, Engineering, and Medicine published a comprehensive report, concluding that there is "substantial evidence" that cannabis is an effective treatment for chronic pain in adults.[3]

Marijuana seems to work especially well when dealing with neuropathic pain, which results from damage to the central nervous system and includes a wide range of conditions such as diabetic neuropathy, shingles, and nerve damage caused by injury or surgery. Pain resulting from chemotherapy and radiation also falls under the umbrella of neuropathic pain, as does central pain syndrome, which can be caused by multiple sclerosis, a stroke, or Parkinson's disease.

Sativex (also known by its generic name, Nabiximols) is a pharmaceutical cannabinoid that contains equal parts THC and CBD. Canada and Israel have approved Sativex for managing neuropathic pain in adult patients suffering from multiple sclerosis, as well for patients who have advanced cancer and are experiencing pain that's not alleviated by opioids. Interestingly, Sativex, which is an oral spray, also contains a handful of terpenes.[4]

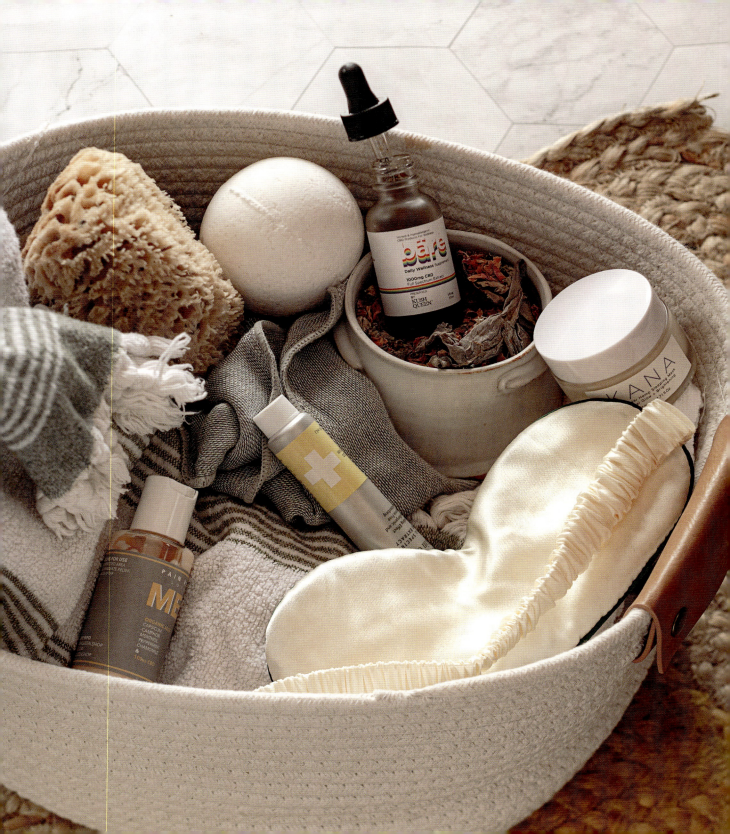

Spasticity

Spasticity is a condition where muscles are continuously contracting, causing stiffness, muscle spasms, and sometimes pain; it is a common symptom of both multiple sclerosis and cerebral palsy, though it may also be caused by a traumatic brain injury (TBI) or spinal cord injury. The science suggesting that cannabis can help alleviate spasticity in MS patients is strong. The same 2017 report from the National Academy of Sciences, Engineering, and Medicine that concluded that cannabis could help with chronic pain stated that there is "substantial evidence" that oral cannabinoids are an effective treatment for improving patient-reported spasticity in MS patients.[5] Currently twenty-five countries have approved Sativex for treating spasticity related to MS.

Bizarrely, the US has yet to approve Sativex for anything.

Nausea

It's no secret that cannabis reduces nausea, making it perfect for patients who are going through chemotherapy. In fact, in 1985, the FDA approved cannabinoid drugs Nabilone and Dronabinol for combating nausea and vomiting associated with chemo in patients who failed to respond adequately to conventional anti-nausea treatments.

More recently, an animal study published in *The British Journal of Pharmacology* in 2013 showed that THCA, the nonpsychoactive precursor to THC, might be more potent at treating nausea than THC. Preclinical studies have also hinted that CBD shows promise in treating nausea. More research on THCA, CBD, and CBDA is needed, but the evidence strongly supports the anti-nausea benefits of cannabis.

Decreased Appetite

If you've smoked pot or ingested it in any form you may be all too familiar with the concept of "the munchies"—I certainly am. But for people with chronic diseases that cause appetite loss or cachexia (a weakening and wasting of the body), THC's appetite-stimulating qualities can be a lifesaver, or, at the very least, a life-extender.

There is sound evidence showing that cannabis effectively promotes weight gain in HIV/AIDS patients. However, current studies on cannabis's ability to promote weight gain with cancer patients and anorexia nervosa patients have been inconclusive.[6] Luckily, these disappointing results don't mean that cannabis won't spur the appetite of cancer and anorexia nervosa patients; they simply point to our need for better-quality, placebo-controlled trials that use the right amount of cannabis. Some recent trials administered only 2.5 milligrams of THC twice a day, leading researchers to conclude that higher doses of THC (along with some CBD to help control potential side effects) might be effective.

As cannabis researcher Michael Backes explains in his book, *Cannabis Pharmacy*, cannabis likely stimulates the nucleus accumbens, an area of the midbrain that causes overeating and increases food palatability.[7] As scientists learn more about the endocannabinoid system, which, among other things, regulates appetite, we'll likely develop a better understanding of the mysterious munchies.

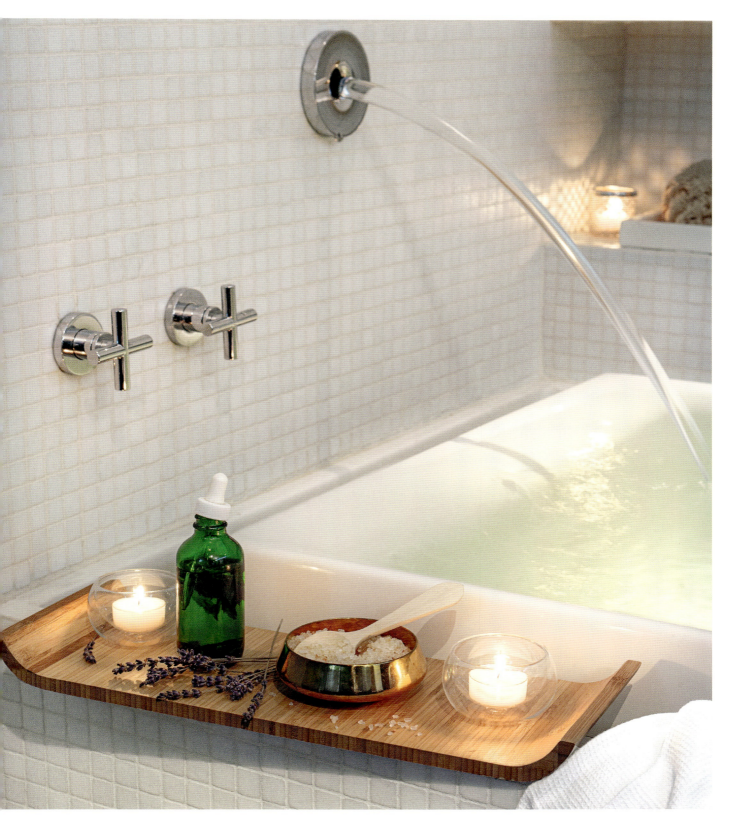

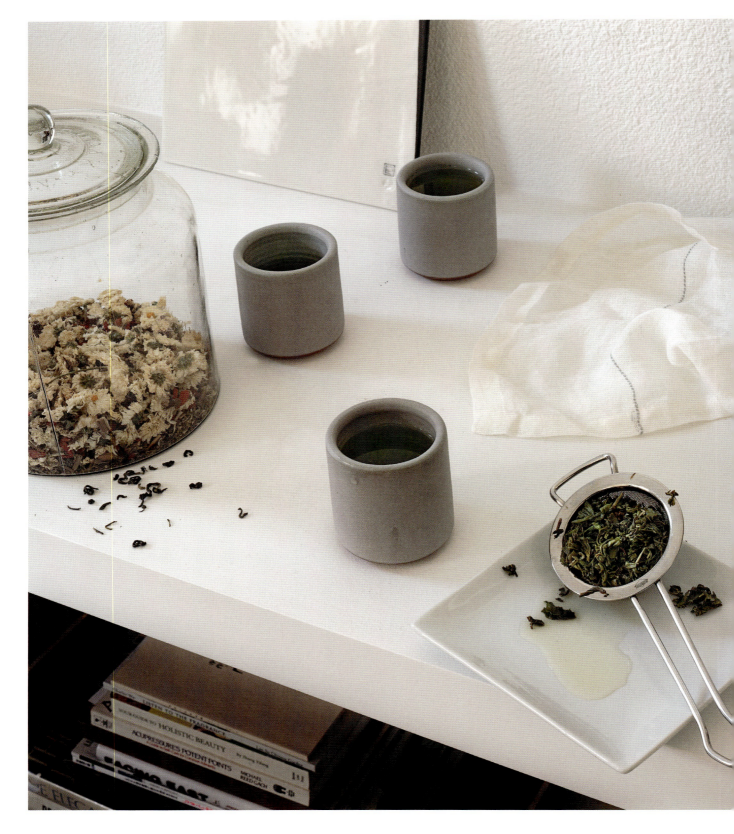

Epilepsy

According to Dr. Ethan Russo, director of research and development for the International Cannabis and Cannabinoids Institute, cannabis has been used to treat epilepsy since ancient times. "If ancient Assyrian sources referring to 'hand of ghost' are considered credible, this relationship may span four millennia," Russo wrote, in a review for *Epilepsy & Behavior*.[8]

It has taken modern science quite a while to catch up. The FDA's approval of Epidiolex in 2018 (a 100 percent CBD medication to treat two rare pediatric seizure disorders) marked a turning point.

Clearly, there were very high-quality, randomized, and controlled trials run to study CBD's ability to reduce seizures, since the FDA sets a very high bar for approval of any pharmaceutical.

But what about THC?

Though THC shows promise in reducing seizures—as does THC combined with CBD—most of the studies to date have been small and of poor quality. In its 2017 report, the National Academies of Sciences, Engineering, and Medicine determined that there was insufficient evidence to either support or refute the conclusion that cannabinoids provide an effective treatment for epilepsy, but this was before the results of the Epidiolex trials had been published.

That said, extensive observations from practitioners have shown that much lower doses of CBD, when used with a small amount of THC, THCA, and even linalool (a terpene that may have anticonvulsant properties), help to reduce seizures.[9] Clearly, more rigorous randomized controlled trials are needed to understand whether THC alone or THC combined with CBD (and possibly THCA and linalool) can significantly reduce seizures.

Insomnia and
Other Sleep Disorders

Some people seem to sleep better after they ingest a little cannabis; others stay up late into the night, their thoughts racing. While this contradiction may be due to differences in each person's unique endocannabinoid system, it may also have to do with which strain you are consuming or how sensitive you are to THC.

A recent retrospective case study of seventy-two adults presenting with anxiety and poor sleep habits found that CBD alone helped reduce anxiety and initially improved sleep in adults.[10] Though CBD is known to decrease anxiety, it is not as effective as a sleep aid and can actually be stimulating to some people. Interestingly, CBD's effectiveness as a sleep aid does improve when combined with THC.

Also, consider which terpenes are dominant in the strain you're selecting. Some strains contain terpenes such as myrcene or linalool that have sedating effects; others contain terpenes such as limonene or pinene that deliver alertness and mental clarity. (See Chapter 2 for more on terpenes.)

Even the National Academy of Sciences, Engineering, and Medicine admits that cannabis could play a role in treating sleep disorders and says there is "moderate evidence" that cannabinoids are an effective treatment for sleep disturbances, particularly those associated with sleep apnea, fibromyalgia, chronic pain, and multiple sclerosis.

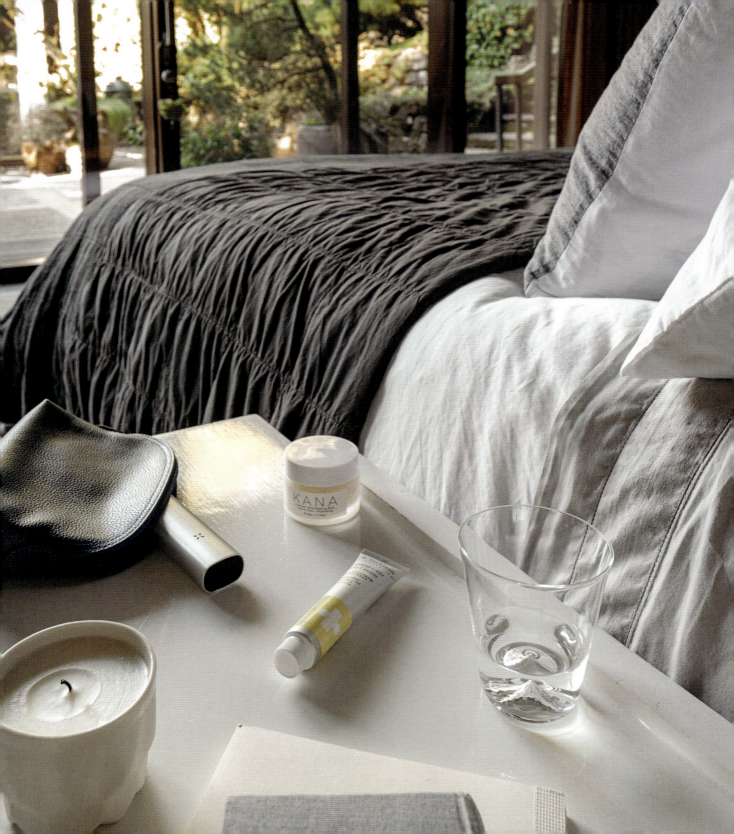

Rheumatoid Arthritis

One thing we know for sure is that cannabis has powerful anti-inflammatory properties. Nowhere is this better demonstrated than with rheumatoid arthritis (RA), an autoimmune disease characterized by serious inflammation of a joint's interior lining. RA's severe inflammation causes chronic pain, and while we know there's strong evidence documenting cannabis's pain-relieving properties, there is also ample evidence establishing the anti-inflammatory effects of cannabis and hemp.

The makers of Sativex had a hunch that their drug would work on RA, and in 2016, they published the results of their study. The thirty-one RA patients randomly selected to take Sativex showed a statistically significant reduction in pain caused by movement and activity, as well as pain felt while at rest or asleep, when compared to the twenty-seven RA patients who received a placebo.[11]

However, this was a small study, and to date it's the only study that's been done to interrogate the relationship between cannabis and RA in humans. In a 2019 review called "Joints for Joints: Cannabinoids in the Treatment of Rheumatoid Arthritis," scientists from the University Hospital Düsseldorf in Germany looked at how cannabinoids cause a decrease in inflammation by activating CB2 receptors. Leading scientists in the field now propose that future studies on RA focus on these CB2 receptors and other mechanisms.[12] In the meantime, the lack of large, high-quality studies hasn't kept patients with RA from using cannabis to treat their symptoms.

Interestingly, the latest science is showing that THCA, the nonpsychoactive precursor of THC, may be more effective for treating skin inflammation than even THC.[13] Hopefully in the coming years, more research will be done to help us determine which combination of cannabinoids is best for treating RA.

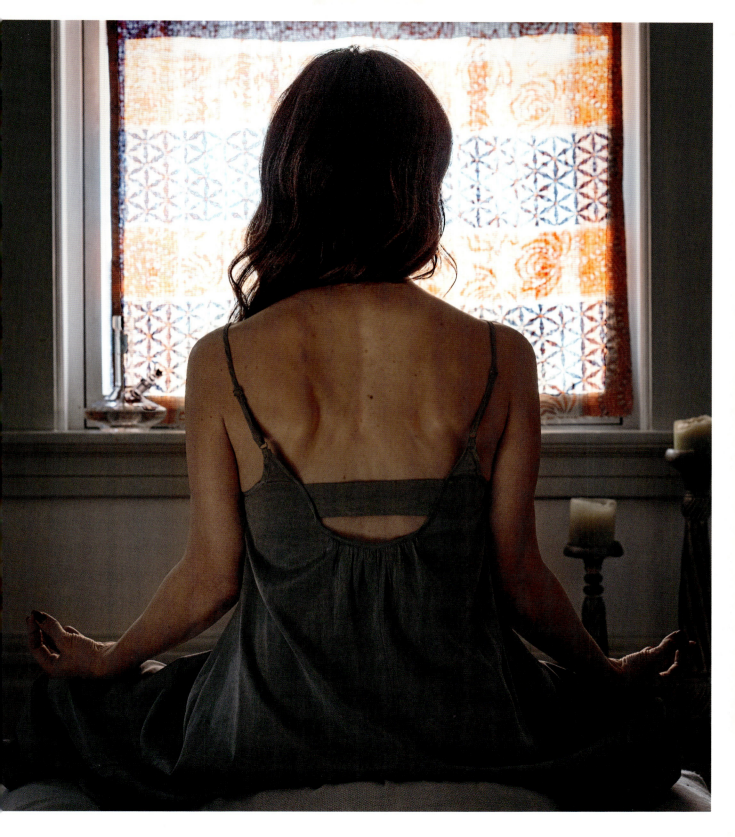

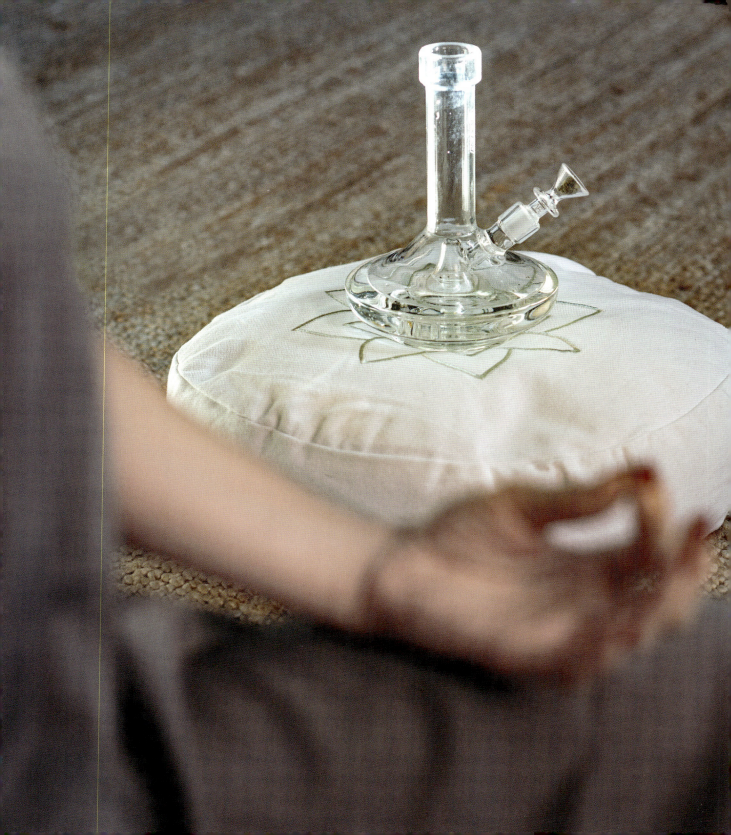

Anxiety Disorders

Anxiety disorders include generalized anxiety disorder (GAD), panic attacks, and social anxiety. Though post-traumatic stress disorder (PTSD) and obsessive-compulsive disorder (OCD) are often associated with anxiety, *The Diagnostic and Statistical Manual of Mental Disorders* no longer classifies them as such.

While cannabis seems to decrease anxiety in some, it may actually increase anxious feelings in others. This could be due to dosage; higher doses tend to trigger anxiety and sometimes even paranoia in susceptible individuals—or it may have to do with each person's unique endocannabinoid system. It's also possible that the mind-set of the user and the setting in which the cannabis is consumed have a bearing on what effects marijuana will have on a consumer.

While there have been a few randomized controlled studies done that show that synthetic THC medications like Dronabinal and Nabilone are capable of delivering a greater short-term reduction in anxiety than a placebo, in truth, CBD shows far more promise as an antianxiety treatment than THC.

Several studies have shown that people who took CBD prior to public speaking experienced reduced levels of anxiety.[14] A small study published in the *Brazilian Journal of Medical and Biological Research* showed that plasma cortisol levels decreased significantly when people took 300 milligrams of oral CBD as opposed to a placebo.[15] High blood cortisol levels are a sign of stress and anxiety. In a 2015 review of CBD as a potential treatment for anxiety disorders, a group of researchers at NYU wrote, "Evidence from human studies strongly supports the potential for CBD as a treatment for anxiety disorders."[16] More recent research, including a case series published in 2019, showed that a majority of 103 adults with anxiety and poor sleep habits reported significantly reduced anxiety scores after taking 25–75 milligrams of CBD per day in capsule form.[17] Overall, the general consensus is that CBD is a safe, nontoxic way to reduce anxiety.

Because of its anti-inflammatory properties, and the way the plant interacts with our endocannabinoid system, cannabis can improve the symptoms of many diseases and chronic conditions. Research is ongoing on cannabis as a treatment for ALS, Alzheimer's disease, various autoimmune diseases, cancer/glioma, diabetes, irritable bowel syndrome, and Parkinson's disease. And while there are plenty of anecdotal reports showing successful treatment of these conditions using cannabis, right now there isn't enough scientific evidence to conclusively say whether the plant is an effective treatment for these diseases. Let's hope the scientific community continues to study the possibly life-changing effects of the cannabis plant.

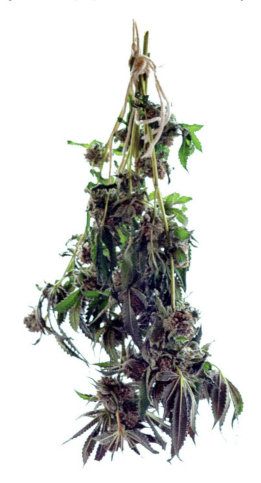

Q & A

WITH RACHEL KNOX, MD

CO-FOUNDER OF THE AMERICAN CANNABINOID CLINICS

It's not easy to find an MD who is well versed in cannabis science and the medical benefits of cannabis. In Oregon, one family of doctors stands out from the rest: the Knox family. Dad David, mom Janice, and daughters Jessica and Rachel collectively launched the American Cannabinoid Clinics in 2017. Though they have a brick-and-mortar clinic in Portland, where David Knox is the primary doctor, most of the Knox Docs practice telemedicine, which allows them to counsel people worldwide. They also spend a lot of time on the road speaking about cannabis and the endocannabinoid system at anti-aging conferences, cannabis science symposiums, and even ancient-nutrition gatherings.

The family recently launched the Advent Academy, a virtual place of higher learning where doctors, nurses, and other healthcare professionals can advance their cannabis education. "All healthcare professionals should be involved in the cannabis conversation," says Rachel Knox, 37. I talked to Rachel Knox about the family's business, and the importance of nutrition in balancing the endocannabinoid system.

ꙮ Do you still see patients at the Sellwood clinic in Portland?

Some people—baby boomers and older—are still old-school and want to be seen in person. So, us Portland folk—my dad and I mostly—we tag-team our clinic. It's hard to get leases even though cannabis has been legal here for so long. We were looking for a new Portland office, and we looked for six months—and we don't even touch the plant!

🌿 How do patients find you?

Pediatric patients come to us from referrals from Oregon Health and Science University. They don't want to touch cannabis with a ten-foot pole! Adults find us because they might be googling online—maybe they saw us on the *Megyn Kelly* show or saw my TEDx talk [in Portland in 2019]. We're rogue, through the lens of the conventional system.

🌿 What was your cannabis awakening?

I was a little kid when it was legalized medically. Maybe it's our generation, but I did not have a "come to Jesus moment." My sister and I went to Tufts University School of Medicine, which has a dual degree program with the business school. When we were getting ready to apply to residencies, I thought, "This is so out of alignment with my core values. I'm learning to become a doctor in a sick care system." I wanted to learn about nutrition, botanical medicine. I caught wind of an integrative medicine fellowship in Arizona. The program addressed disease at its root cause.

Meanwhile, my parents were already working with cannabis clinics in Portland. I would take the info they were learning back to my attendants. "There's not enough research," they'd say. By the latter half of my medical residency, everyone knew I wasn't applying to a traditional job. So about six months after I started talking about cannabis, I was like, "That's what I'm going to do." They were like, "She's lost her mind."

🌿 What diseases or conditions does cannabis seem to help most, based on what you've seen in your practice?

We get a lot of cancer patients. When people first come in, we hit them with their endocannabinoid system, nutrition (their first line of defense), and their first medical resource. We have to reframe expectations, because most people see us for cannabis. So when they come to our clinics, they learn how nutrition maintains the ECS and how cannabis can be an adjunct. Most people have more than one disease process: Chronic pain, depression, and anxiety can all be mixed in there. They might have IBS or IBD, plus insomnia, plus arthritis. We also see a lot of autoimmunity.

🌿 **Part of your job is educating patients about what the endocannabinoid system is and how cannabis—in all its many forms—interacts with it. Do most patients already know about the ECS, or do you have to blow their minds with this information?**
Of course not. They're like, "What? I have an endocannabinoid system?" And we're like, "Yeah, you do!"

🌿 **What are your thoughts and theories on full-spectrum cannabis versus pharmaceutical types of cannabis that tend to isolate one cannabinoid (like THC) and not include others? Is full-spectrum always better, and if so, why?**
In the few clinical trials that we have, full-spectrum has been better than isolates. Full-spectrum also has a broader safety profile, and tolerability is higher. The margin of safety is better. With isolates, we see something called the biphasic effect. If you were to graph it, you would see a bell-shaped curve. At low doses you're increasing effect, then there's a point at which you decrease effect and get unwanted side effects. As you get closer to an isolate, that window of tolerability starts to shrink. You won't have the other phytochemicals on board to buffer that isolate. We want people to be using a full-spectrum product.

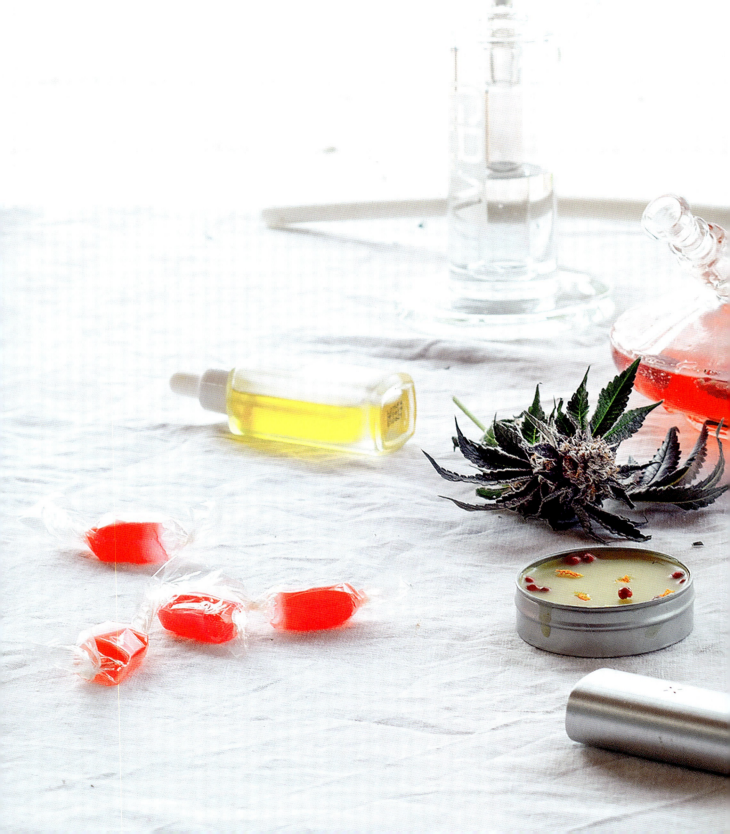

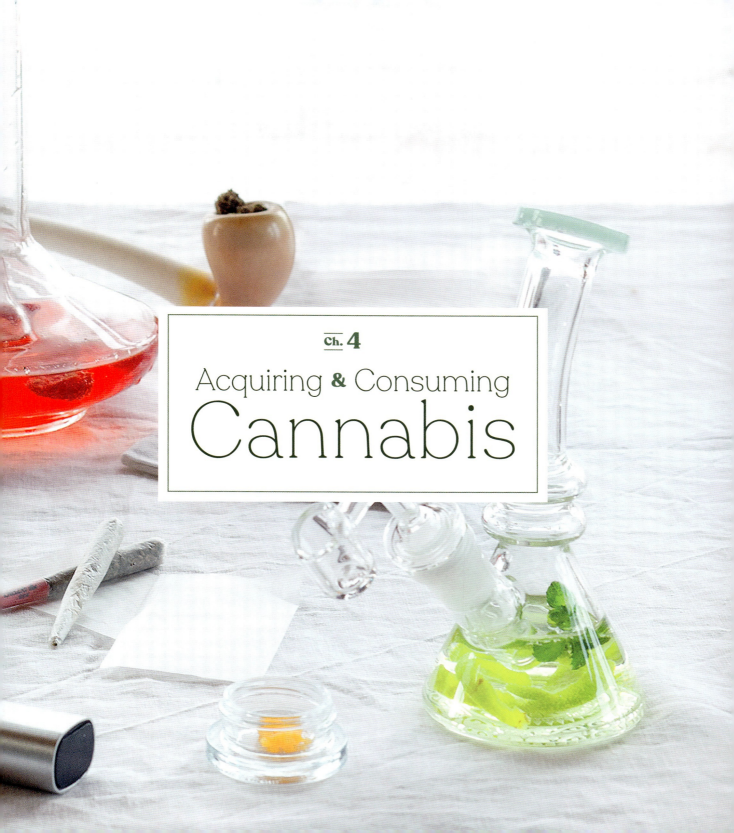

Ch. **4**

Acquiring & Consuming
Cannabis

In this chapter I'll share my favorite strains, both for cooking and for recreational purposes. I'll explore several of the most widely used strains and what makes them tick. I tend to like to cook with what I like to smoke. And truth be told, these days I don't often find many strains I don't like to smoke, which I think speaks to the amazing quality of Oregon cannabis. When my relationship with recreational drugs began, thousands of edibles ago, there were few options. There were a couple of strains of cannabis: Panama Red and Acapulco Gold—and one type of hash that was superstrong and hard to get (Afghani, I think). "Scoring" the cannabis was always an adventure, the kind I hope my kids never engaged in. None of my friends grew weed, and as far as I knew, nobody's parents indulged. A few people had cool parents, but if they partook, they were discreet about it.

The thing I loved most about getting high back then was how much we laughed. My recollection is that 95 percent of the time I spent eating brownies or smoking a joint was a barrel of fun, usually coupled with a few profound insights and a crazy bout of the munchies. I remember there was this pudding you could get from the freezer section at the grocery called Cool 'n Creamy, and I would sit with that container and a spoon and finish the whole thing in one sitting. My friends and I would each get our own—it was such a decadent stoner taste sensation. Today I continue to seek that same sense of pleasure with a container of Kozy Shack pudding, which is also delicious. You could even stir in a little infused oil or butter if you wanted to keep the party going, but not too much. Remember: Less is more. And no, I don't have stock in that company, though I wish I did.

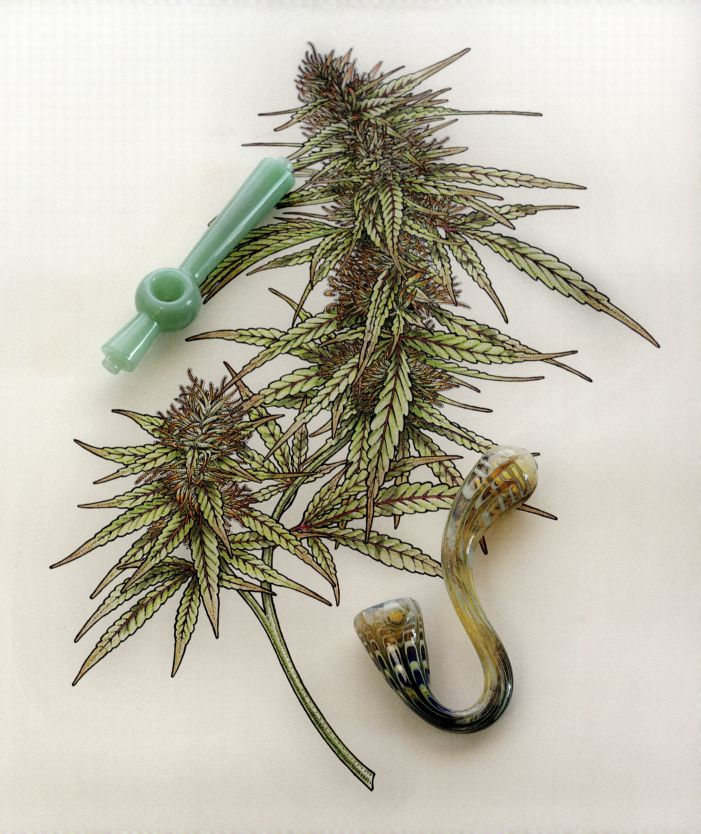

I have no distinct memory of feeling different effects from the different forms of cannabis my friends and I tried; although now, looking back, I think the terpenes were responsible for the occasional death grip of paranoia I experienced. I remember being in my friend Beth's parents' apartment on Johnson Avenue in the Bronx, getting super freaked-out, listening to "Long Black Veil" by The Band on a record player. Eventually I got under the covers in her parents' bed (they were out, obviously) because I was so anxious and paranoid. That was my first seriously unpleasant drug experience. Thankfully, I persevered.

Potency as a Percentage

The potency of cannabis and hemp buds are presented as a percentage of the THC and CBD (and any other cannabinoid) tested/found in the flower. This percentage represents the weight of the amount of the particular cannabinoid in relation to the total weight of the plant material. So for a 20 percent THC bud, that means that 20 percent of the bud's composition is THC. If you weigh that bud and it's 1 gram (and we know that 1 gram = 1,000 milligrams), that would mean that there are 200 milligrams of THC in that bud (1,000 · 0.20 = 200). I think we could write some really fun math problems for those algebra books.

If you're fortunate enough to live in a country in which cannabis is legalized, the dispensaries in these locations are required to provide all the necessary information you need to make informed decisions on what to purchase (test results free of pesticides, percentage of THC, CBD, CBG, etc.), but there is no substitute for taking a puff from a joint or hit on a pipe to help you determine how you feel about a strain. Back in the day, before I invested in a mountain of cannabis for smoking and cooking, I would buy the smallest amount of a strain I could, smoke a tiny bit, and see what I thought. If I liked it, I would buy an ounce, or even a half-ounce to infuse some butter.

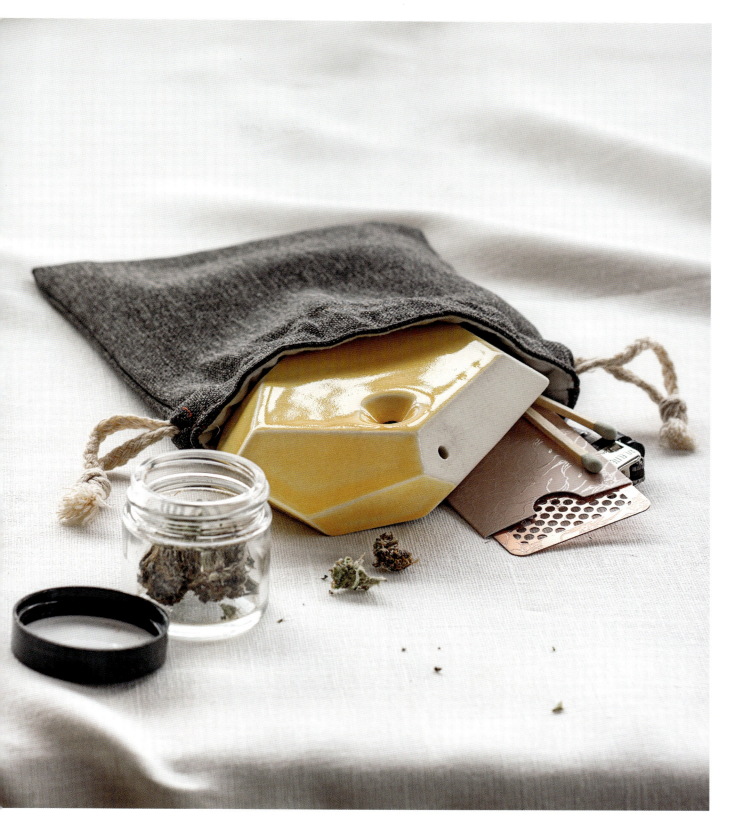

Interestingly, in today's booming marijuana market, making a decision as to which strain you prefer is both much easier and more difficult than ever. And my advice throughout this book will be to look, if you can, at the terpene profiles of the cannabis you are using. Once you are armed with some important basic information on terpenes and cannabinoids, the compounds in cannabis that inform the smell, taste, and effects of the plant, you will be able to pick a strain for the right reasons based on the terpene profile, the cannabinoid profile, and the potency. While many people still use the basic terms "indica" and "sativa" to differentiate between strains, this practice is quickly falling by the wayside, which is resulting in a fair amount of confusion among consumers. Since there is no governing, FDA-like body that controls the entire marijuana industry, a plant may be named anything at all, and strains can be crossbred and plant genetics can be altered. In the new pot landscape, the best way to choose the strain that is right for you is to choose based on terpene and cannabinoid profiles, which were discussed in depth in Chapter 2.

The whole indica vs. sativa thing is in the middle of quite an upheaval. Due to crossbreeding and our changing understanding of the underlying genetics, using that terminology will get you no more than the shape of the plant. Knowing the terpene and cannabinoid profiles is like knowing the science, and on that you can rely. This is not fake news. While these descriptions of indica and sativa strains may have profiles that sound right and easy to understand, there is more information needed to make an informed choice.

This is an interesting moment. A few years from now, the terms "indica" and "sativa" may be a distant memory. I have been speaking with chemists and cultivators who see the change coming quickly, and several companies are no longer using indica and sativa. But relax, the transition will be gradual. For terms so *baked* into the industry and culture, it's hard to imagine them going away completely.

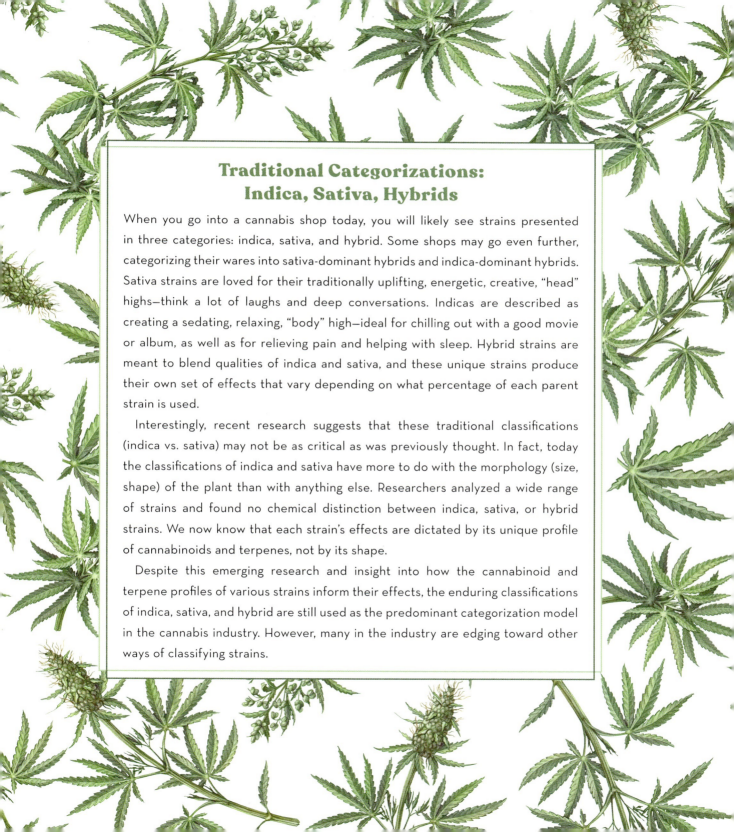

Traditional Categorizations:
Indica, Sativa, Hybrids

When you go into a cannabis shop today, you will likely see strains presented in three categories: indica, sativa, and hybrid. Some shops may go even further, categorizing their wares into sativa-dominant hybrids and indica-dominant hybrids. Sativa strains are loved for their traditionally uplifting, energetic, creative, "head" highs—think a lot of laughs and deep conversations. Indicas are described as creating a sedating, relaxing, "body" high—ideal for chilling out with a good movie or album, as well as for relieving pain and helping with sleep. Hybrid strains are meant to blend qualities of indica and sativa, and these unique strains produce their own set of effects that vary depending on what percentage of each parent strain is used.

Interestingly, recent research suggests that these traditional classifications (indica vs. sativa) may not be as critical as was previously thought. In fact, today the classifications of indica and sativa have more to do with the morphology (size, shape) of the plant than with anything else. Researchers analyzed a wide range of strains and found no chemical distinction between indica, sativa, or hybrid strains. We now know that each strain's effects are dictated by its unique profile of cannabinoids and terpenes, not by its shape.

Despite this emerging research and insight into how the cannabinoid and terpene profiles of various strains inform their effects, the enduring classifications of indica, sativa, and hybrid are still used as the predominant categorization model in the cannabis industry. However, many in the industry are edging toward other ways of classifying strains.

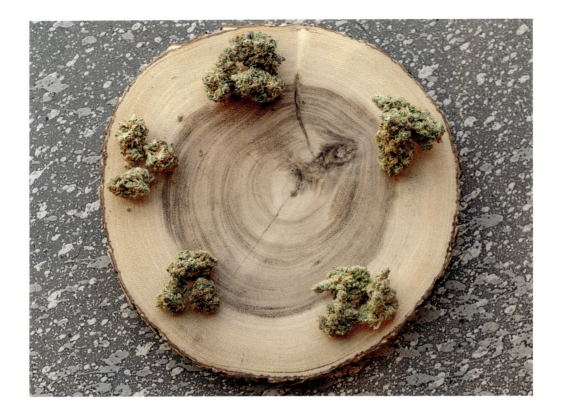

Indicas are well-loved for their ability to offer a relaxing body high and to treat medical issues including pain, spasms, anxiety, nausea, and sleep problems. Strain names have gotten pretty out-there over time, with names like Zookies and Ice Cream Cake. These names, while fun, often have little or nothing to do with the genetic makeup of the plant. The amount of THC and CBD content is different for every strain, so it's important to make an informed decision before selecting your strain. This will allow you to have a more controlled experience.

Environmental factors like temperature, sunlight, soil type, and food/nutrients will also impact the ultimate output and effects of a plant. This is why strains can vary so wildly from grower to grower and from harvest to harvest. So don't be surprised if the OG Kush from one grower is not quite the same as the OG Kush from another. We hope you will find this guide helpful in your search for the perfect strain.

A Guide to Common Strains

9 POUND HAMMER

Indica | THC: 14–23% | CBD: 0.0–0.25%

9 Pound Hammer was bred as a cross between Jack the Ripper, Hell's OG, and fruity Gooberry. It is an impressive strain useful for pain and stress relief that also comes with a pleasant uptick in creativity and focus. 9 Pound Hammer is known to help spur users on in artistic endeavors.

FLAVOR PROFILE: This plant's diverse lineage results in a sweet mix of flavors with hints of earth and citrus.

MEDICINAL USES: Anxiety disorder, depression, insomnia, muscle spasms, nausea, and pain.

BERRY WHITE

Indica | THC: 19–25% | CBD: 0.3%

As an offspring strain of the legendary Blueberry and White Widow plants, Berry White will deliver a strong high leading to an upbeat afternoon of conversation and creativity. Expect effects such as euphoria and relaxation mixed with a desire to "get up and go."

FLAVOR PROFILE: A mix of soul berry and woody oak, with an aroma to match.

MEDICINAL USES: Ease from depression, insomnia, pain, and stress while stimulating appetite.

BLUE DREAM

Hybrid | THC: 17–24% | CBD: 0.1–0.2%

A great-tasting hybrid, Blue Dream produces full-body relaxation with a calm sense of euphoria. Originating in California, it is increasingly popular on the West Coast. Both new and longtime fans of Blue Dream have noted the strain's enjoyable level of effects, which bring a relaxed but swift relief to symptoms such as pain or depression, and do so without heavy sedative side effects. Blue Dream is a solid choice for those seeking a strain suitable for daytime activity.

FLAVOR PROFILE: Sweet, herbal, fruity, and floral with notes of blueberry, mango, and vanilla.

MEDICINAL USES: Anorexia/cachexia, depression, migraines, nausea, pain, sleep disorders, and stress.

BLUEBERRY DIESEL

Hybrid | THC: 13–23% | CBD: 0%

A cross between Blueberry and Sour Diesel, this strain has a powerful blueberry aroma. This calming strain is a mixture of mental and physical relaxation, allowing for a three-to-four-hour respite from what stresses you out.

FLAVOR PROFILE: A strong scent of blueberry, giving off a fruity and tangy aroma that results in a fruity, pleasantly bitter taste.

MEDICINAL USES: Anxiety disorder, appetite stimulant, depression, pain, and migraines.

BLUEBERRY MUFFIN

Hybrid | THC: 20–22% | CBD: 0.4%

The blueberry aroma in this strain is a true showstopper. It's kind of amazing how strong the flavor is. The strain is great for pain management, and although it is extremely calming, there is no couch-lock, so you are good to go about your day while feeling relaxed and happy.

FLAVOR PROFILE: Sweet and fresh berry flavors mix with just a hint of earthy skunkiness.

MEDICINAL USES: Energizing yet relaxing, this mood lifter gives users feelings of euphoria and ease from anxiety, migraines, PTSD, sleep disorders, and stress while acting as an appetite enhancer.

BUBBA KUSH

Indica | THC: 14–22% | CBD: 0.0–0.01%

Choose Bubba Kush and you will be thoroughly chilled out and relaxed. One of the most sedating strains, expect relief from anxiety and depression. Look for this strain to offer both feelings of euphoria and sleepiness.

FLAVOR PROFILE: Sweet, herbal, and floral notes interwoven with hints of chocolate, coffee, and nuts.

MEDICINAL USES: Ease from depression, insomnia, pain, and stress while quite an appetite stimulant.

G-13

Indica | THC: 22–24% | CBD: 0.17%

G-13 has a legend nearly unmatched in the cannabis world. According to some, in the mid-twentieth century, the CIA and the FBI set out to gather the best marijuana strains from the best growers in the world. Following this collection, the two organizations chose the best hybrids and crossbred them, leading to the creation of G-13. Though the legend may not be true, this strain is definitely worth trying. Expect a powerful body high and serious couch-lock.

FLAVOR PROFILE: Earthy with hints of mint and musk; a pleasing combination of sweet and spicy.

MEDICINAL USES: Anorexia/cachexia, anxiety disorder, arthritis, depression, lack of appetite, migraines, nausea, sleep disorders, and stress.

Pot Talk

The term "couch-lock" describes the tendency, when high, to not want to move or exert any energy or the feeling of not having the energy or motivation to leave the couch. It is often associated with the terpene myrcene, the most predominant terpene in cannabis, and the terpene most commonly linked with traditional indica strains.

GODFATHER OG

Indica | THC: 25–28% | CBD: 0.5%

Likely to be a potent strain, this sedating indica will be sure to reduce your stress and keep you feeling deeply relaxed. Often referred to as the Don of All OGs, this flower is bred from XXX OG and Alpha OG. With THC numbers that are quite high, you can look forward to relaxation and a peaceful night's sleep.

FLAVOR PROFILE: Strong notes of pine and earth, with hints of grape popping through.

MEDICINAL USES: Ease from depression, headaches, insomnia, and pain.

> ### Pot Talk
> Using the term "OG" in strain names can refer to a couple of things: either "ocean grown" (cannabis cultivated near the ocean or in a state on the coast) or "original gangster."

GRANDDADDY PURPLE

Indica | THC: 17–23% | CBD: 0.1–0.3%

Granddaddy Purple (GDP) is an easily distinguishable plant known for its white tips nestled on a background of deep purple flowers, hence the name. Also well-known for its room-filling aroma of berry and fruitiness, GDP will help you reach a deep state of relaxation and offers a stress-free "sesh." The Granddaddy delivers a strong effect both to the body and the mind, resulting in

a feeling of euphoria as well as a sense of physical calm and well-being.

FLAVOR PROFILE: A tropical, sweet strain with notes of berry and grape.

MEDICINAL USES: Ease from pain, headaches, insomnia, migraines, nausea, Alzheimer's disease, and Parkinson's disease.

GHOST TRAIN HAZE

Sativa | THC: 18–25% | CBD: 0.0–0.01%

Ghost Train Haze is a cross between Ghost OG and Neville's Wreck. This strain is a popular one and has won several awards for its strong concentration of THC. While the strong concentration of THC is enough to ease most pain and depression, if you are a user prone to anxiety, stay away.

FLAVOR PROFILE: Earthy with notes of citrus and berry.

MEDICINAL USES: Ease from depression, fatigue, headaches, pain, and stress.

ISLAND SWEET SKUNK

Sativa | THC: 18–20% | CBD: 0.0–0.01%

Island Sweet Skunk is an energizing strain with antianxiety and anti-inflammatory properties. It also helps with nerve pain, migraines, arthritis, and gastrointestinal disorders. You will experience energizing, uplifting, and euphoric effects while noticing a decrease in stress and aches and pains.

FLAVOR PROFILE: Sweet, skunky, and tropical.

MEDICINAL USES: Anxiety, arthritis, fatigue, migraines, nausea, pain, PTSD, and stress.

IRISH CREAM

Indica | THC: 14–20% | CBD: 1.0%

This is a strain meant for nighttime use. It is sedating and is best used when you're planning a warm and cozy night in front of the television. This strain originated in Ireland, and that's cool. The strain helps to alleviate muscle aches and pains, both temporary and chronic.

FLAVOR PROFILE: A fruity and sweet aroma with a skunky undertone. Accompanied by a standout flavor of coffee and cream.

MEDICINAL USES: Arthritis, anxiety, depression, headache, insomnia, lupus, and pain.

LAMB'S BREAD

Sativa | THC: 16–21% | CBD: 0.0–0.01%

Also known as Lamb's Breath, this energetic and uplifting sativa is said to have been one of Bob Marley's favorite strains. You will feel uplifted, wide awake, and in a super good mood. This strain is used to deal with mental health issues such as anxiety, depression, and bipolar disorder. Some users have noted that Lamb's Bread can lead to feelings of paranoia, so tread carefully when trying this strain for the first time.

FLAVOR PROFILE: A pungent aroma and earthy, woody taste.

MEDICINAL USES: Ease from ADD/ADHD, anxiety, depression, dizziness, dry eyes, dry mouth, fatigue, headaches, paranoia, and stress.

LAUGHING BUDDHA

Sativa | THC: 18–20% | CBD: 0.0–0.01%

Laughing Buddha is a cross between strains from Thailand and Jamaica. A super-fun strain that leads to feelings of happiness and giggles, the high from Laughing Buddha comes on quickly, and there are occasionally moments where your balance may be a bit off. This is a delightful strain that will make you feel playful and positive.

FLAVOR PROFILE: A pungent mix of spicy, herbal, and earthy flavors.

MEDICINAL USES: Ease from depression, anxiety, fatigue, and stress.

PEZ

Indica | THC: 12–27% | CBD: 0.0–0.01%

Though considered a somewhat sedating strain, Pez offers users relaxation and pain management without a strong couch-lock experience. People indulging in Pez will be left feeling happy, uplifted, focused, and pain free. The high THC does not seem to induce paranoia! Pez is a perfect fit for beginners.

FLAVOR PROFILE: A strain with a sweet aroma and taste of berry and citrus.

MEDICINAL USES: Relief from anxiety disorder, depression, pain, and paranoia.

PB SOUFFLÉ

Indica | THC: 19–21% | CBD: 0.0–0.01%

This strain, with a creamy peanut butter aroma, offers a euphoric high along with strong, relaxing vibes. This is the strain for you if you're looking for a relaxing night in.

FLAVOR PROFILE: Resinous, earthy, and nutty with tones of peanut butter.

MEDICINAL USES: Depression, relief from eye pressure, headaches, glaucoma, inflammation, and insomnia.

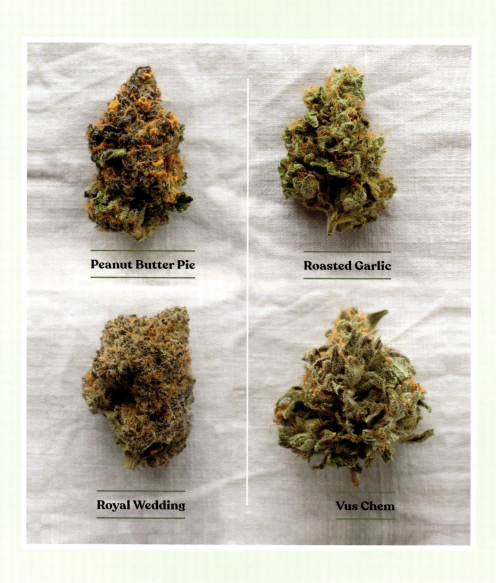

Peanut Butter Pie

Roasted Garlic

Royal Wedding

Vus Chem

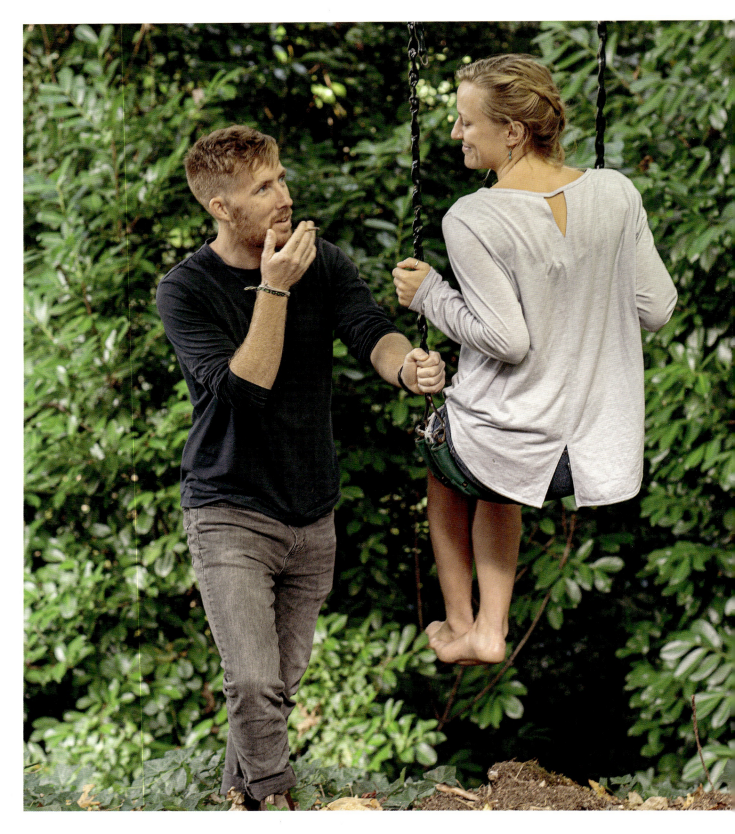

Delivery Methods

There are a variety of ways to consume cannabis, from smoking a joint, to eating an edible, to inserting a suppository (yup, that's a thing) or rubbing on a pain-relieving topical. Each option has its own set of effects, benefits, and constraints. And since everyone processes cannabis differently, you should be aware that what works for one person might not work for you. You should also be aware by now that not all cannabis is the same. The cannabinoid and terpene profile of a strain will certainly influence what effects you will experience, as will the amount you consume and the way you consume it.

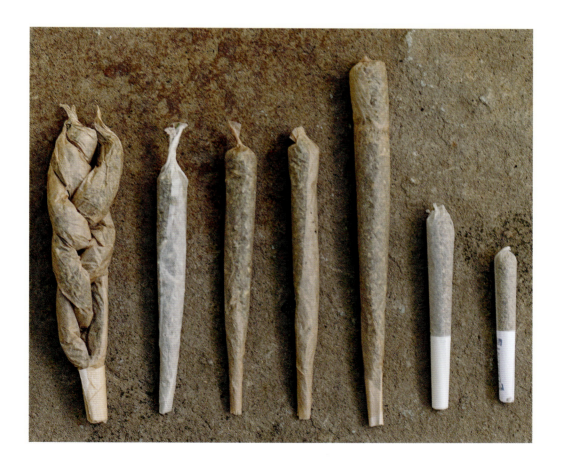

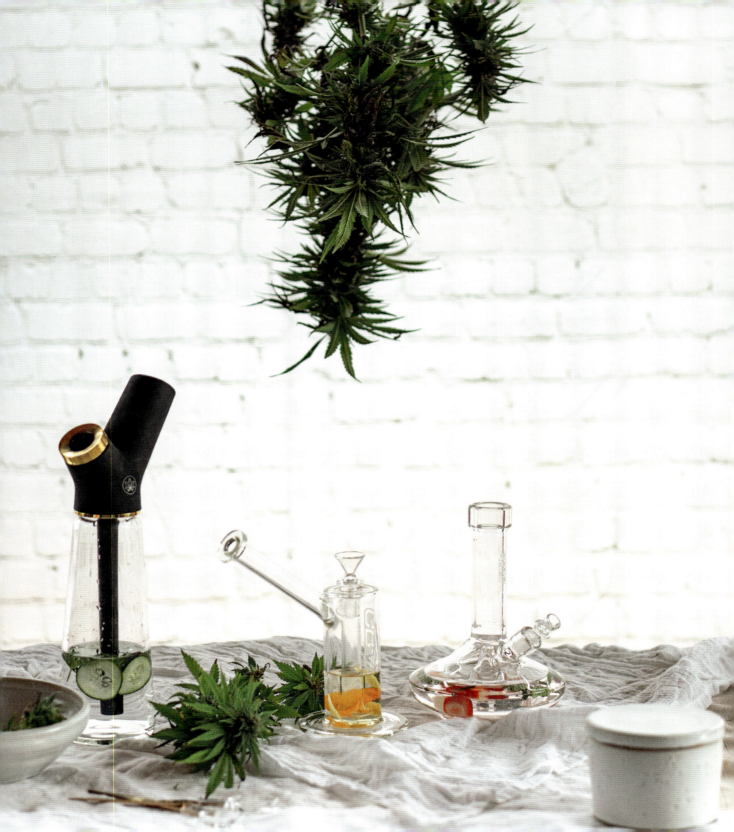

SMOKING

Smoking is pretty straightforward—you light a joint (or bong or pipe) and inhale (from the end that is not burning; believe me, that is not a mistake I will be repeating). My relationship with cannabis started with a joint. A joint, if it's possible you don't know, is a rolled cannabis cigarette, which can also contain resin-based forms of cannabis like kief or hash. Joints, also called splifs, jays, blunts, reefer, doobie, sticks, and a bunch of other names, take effect almost instantly. These effects can last anywhere from a half hour to a few hours. Some people take a hit from a joint every few minutes, while others, like my brother, Fred, take a couple of hits every few hours.

Pipes and bongs are another popular way to smoke. You don't need any rolling papers or special skills; you just need to put some ground cannabis in the bowl of the pipe and light it up. Some bongs have a spot for adding water, which helps to cool the smoke before you inhale. When I was in college, we used to smoke with a bong that was filled with wine. I think maybe people drank the wine after a "sesh," which sounds absolutely disgusting.

The bummer about pipes and bongs is in the upkeep. If you want to continue having a pleasant pipe experience, you need to clean the device at least once a week. Friends of mine clean their pipes or bongs every day. The preferred cleaning method seems to be using a mixture of coarse salt and alcohol. If you let your pipe or bong soak for a bit in this mixture and then give it a good rub with a cloth or towel, it will be clean and good as new.

> ### Pot Talk
> A splif is also occasionally filled with some amount of tobacco. In Jamaica, the word "splif" is used to refer to a very large joint.

VAPING

One of the most popular forms of inhaling cannabis is through vaporization, or vaping. Vaporizing involves heating the cannabis, either with a heated plate or with heated air, to produce a smokeless vapor. The most common method is with portable handheld vaporizers, often through something called a vape pen, although there are also tabletop vape machines, like the Volcano from Storz and Bickel, the EVO by Vapexhale, and Extreme Q by Arizer.

There are two styles of vaping: You can vape either flower/buds or oil/extracts. While the safety of vaping oil/extracts is currently up for debate, vaping flower/buds, as long as they are free of pesticides, is a lovely way to inhale cannabis. It's a great option for those who want to intake cannabis by inhalation without the smokiness of lighting up a joint, ripping a bong, or firing up a pipe.

Vape pens are portable and battery operated and contain cartridges filled with cannabis oil/extract. There are many different companies that make these pens, and their quality varies greatly. You should be picky and choose a pen that accommodates top-quality oil and offers as much information as possible on the product you are ingesting. When the oil or extract is placed in a cartridge, and the cartridge is inserted into the vape pen, a battery inside the pen ignites the cartridge and creates the vapor that you inhale. You can buy multiple cartridges to ensure you have more available when one cartridge runs out of goodness. A vape pen has certain qualities that recommend it over old-fashioned smoking. A pen is portable, discreet, and virtually odorless unless you buy a purposefully scented cartridge. This allows you to take your vape pen with you wherever you go. It also allows you to more closely control your dosage and to pace the amount of cannabis you inhale. Some even allow you to adjust the temperature of the vapor you're inhaling, making for a more customized experience. Vape pens were under heavy scrutiny during the writing of this book. Several states have banned vape pens at some level due to a rash of illnesses and deaths linked to vaping oil/extracts. The root cause of these illnesses is unknown

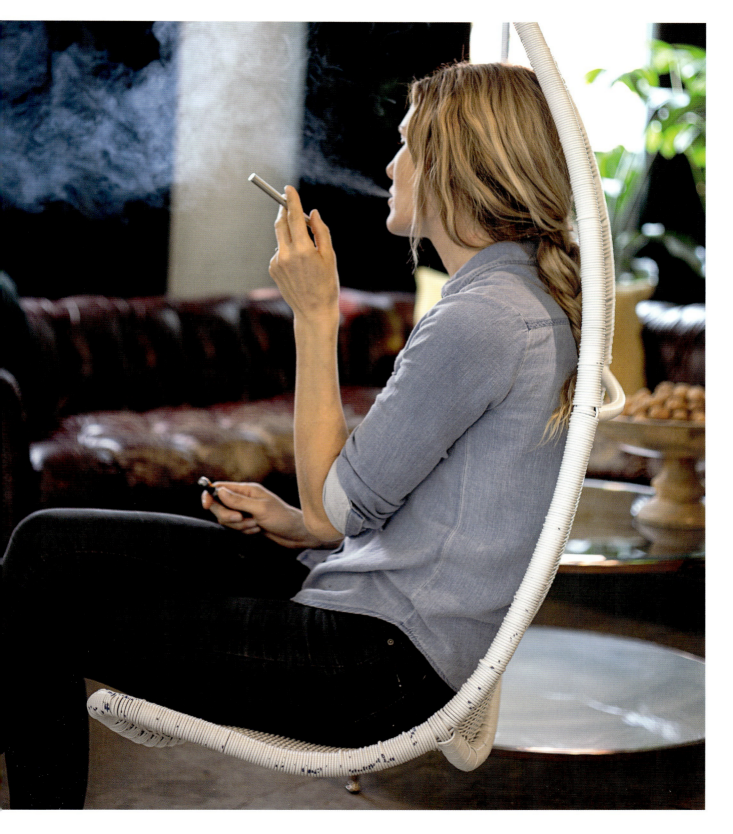

at this time, but the prevailing theories are around black-market products being produced with added thinners like vitamin E acetate, which are harmful when inhaled into the lungs, and cheap vape pens that may be releasing harmful chemicals when heated. If you are going to vape, be sure you are confident in the product and the quality standards of the producer.

DABBING

I have mixed feelings about this method of getting high. Dabbing is done by heating concentrated cannabis products known commonly as shatter or wax. These concentrated products contain huge percentages of THC, which makes dabbing quite intense—almost like extreme vaping. The first time I dabbed I was having a party at my house on the Willamette River. It was a super-cool mix of people, all of whom were pretty serious cannabis users. They offered me a dab, and being the wonderful hostess that I am, I thought saying yes was the polite thing to do. That first time I inhaled, I coughed for twenty minutes, then spent the next forty-five minutes feeling like I was in an astronaut's helmet. I could barely communicate. It wasn't pleasant. That said, I tried it again, and again, and for a while, dabbing became my go-to method for consumption. I now love the way it feels, and it does get me super-high, but the whole experience can feel very uncontrolled. After a couple of months, I decided to stop, because I noticed that joints and edibles were barely affecting me. Dabbing had raised my tolerance so much that it was the only way I could enjoy cannabis. Dabbing is definitely effective, but unless you need a very strong dose, I'd stay away. Or, you know, just dab on your birthday.

TRANSDERMAL PATCH

Transdermal patches are pretty magical. They're like a Band-Aid that you just stick on, and they get you high. No inhaling, no ingesting, just absorption through the skin that enters the bloodstream. They start to take effect pretty quickly, within about ten to fifteen minutes, and their effects can last from eight to twelve hours, depending on their formulation. Some patches have slow-releasing properties that provide relief all day (or all night) long, depending on your needs. This is a great option for folks who cannot smoke or consume edibles.

EDIBLES AND DRINKS

As long as you know the potency of the product you're using, ingesting cannabis is a discreet and delightful way to enjoy marijuana. Edibles provide a body and head high, one that generally comes on slowly and, if you've eaten with caution, will last several hours and leave you relaxed and happy. In my opinion, that's pretty sweet. If you are new to edibles, I recommend starting at a potency of 2 to 5 milligrams THC and wait a full day to assess your reaction to the potency (see the section "Finding Your Dose" later in this chapter for more guidance on finding a dosage that works for you). Everyone has a different tolerance, which has nothing to do with gender or body mass. Each person's body is different, and we all react to edibles in our own way. So start low; better safe than sorry.

CAPSULES

Cannabis-filled capsules are an easy way to enjoy the effects of edibles in pill form. Look for capsules from a good source; you want to buy capsules that are free from pesticides and made from quality oil. Making your own capsule is pretty easy and allows you to tinker with the ideal potency level.

There are small start-up costs associated with making canna-capsules. You will need a capsule machine and empty capsules. These can both be found for pretty reasonable prices online or in some health food stores. You can fill the capsules with your infusions or concentrates of choice. I like to use coconut-oil infusions since the oil is easy to work with and I always have some around. Fill the capsules with as much oil as you can or want and store in a cool place.

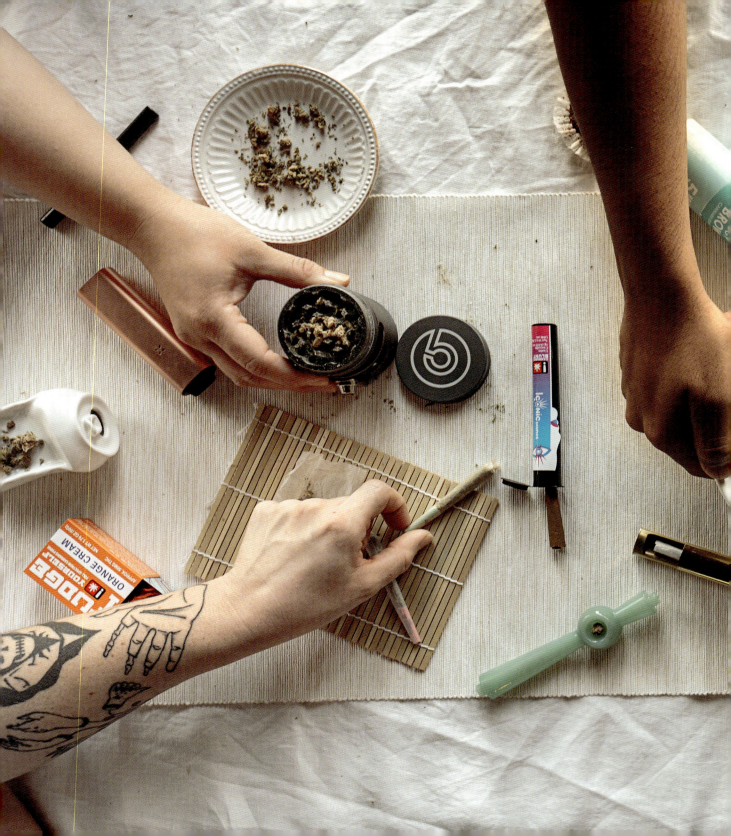

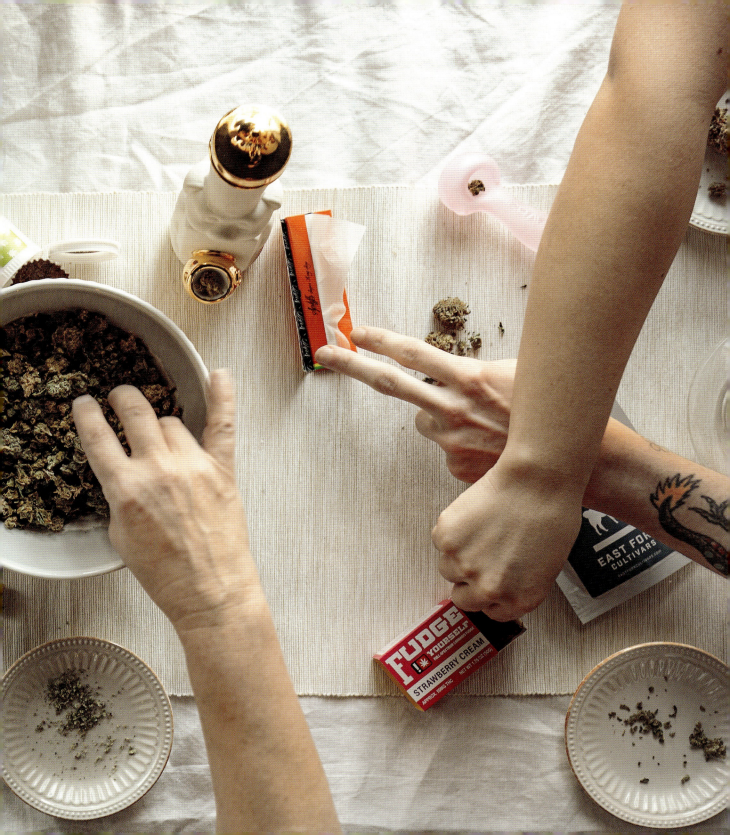

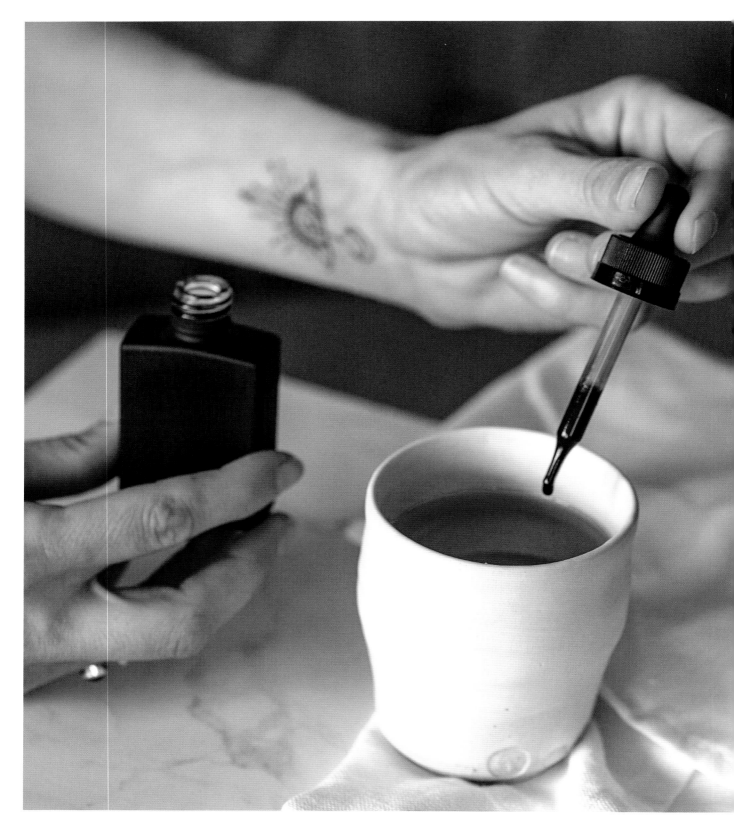

TINCTURES (GREEN OR GOLDEN DRAGON) AND SPRAYS

A cannabis tincture, often referred to as green or golden dragon, is a concentrated liquid made by soaking cannabis in alcohol or glycerin in order to extract the plant's cannabinoids and terpenes. Alcohol acts as an excellent infusion agent, but the taste can leave much to be desired. Some alcohol-based tinctures have a burning sensation that, for me, is a real buzzkill.

I prefer the taste and gentleness of tinctures made with a vegetable glycerin base. Common vegetable glycerin bases are made using soybean, coconut, or palm oils. They do not taste harsh and have a better mouth feel and taste.

Tinctures are typically packaged in a small bottle with a dropper or pipette; occasionally you can find them in a spray bottle. Both packaging options are discreet and easy to use. Simply place a few drops of the tincture under your tongue for quick delivery.

Unlike edibles, the effects of a tincture can be felt quite quickly. You should notice the effects of the tincture between five and fifteen minutes after your initial dosing, with effects lasting anywhere from thirty minutes to two hours. The dosage for tinctures will mirror that of edibles; start with a small level before diving in too far.

Tinctures are a great entry point for both recreational and medical users looking to ease into smokeless methods of use. Plus, they have a long shelf life and should last for quite a while when stored in a cool, dry place.

TOPICALS

Cannabis topicals are infused lotions, oils, balms, and salves that are rubbed on the skin for localized treatment and pain relief. Unlike transdermal patches, they do not get you high. The cannabinoids in topicals do not enter the bloodstream; rather, they permeate the skin/muscle barrier to provide localized relief. When I have muscle pain, there are some products I can rely on for prompt support. After a few minutes, the pain is gone. Cannabis topicals do not offer a cure for pain, but rather a way to manage pain. Honestly, it continues to blow my mind how well these topicals work. I know so many people, including my husband, who swear by topicals and their abilities to relieve pain from sore muscles, inflammation, stress, and tension—as well as their ability to treat psoriasis, arthritis, dermatitis, headaches, and cramping.

SUPPOSITORIES

Though they are not the traditional method of consuming cannabis, both vaginal and anal suppositories offer a fast-acting means for providing pain relief to some of the body's more out-of-the-way spots, and they do so without any psychoactive effects. Rectal suppositories work quickly, spreading the pain-relieving effects of CBD directly into the bloodstream and parceling out to nearby organs within ten to fifteen minutes and lasting for up to eight hours. Vaginal applications have proven to be enormously helpful with gynecological pain associated with endometriosis and painful periods. You may think they're a pain in the ass, but lots of patients have found relief through cannabis suppositories.

Types of Concentrates/Extracts

BHO. Short for "butane hash oil," this concentrate is made from butane extractions. If you go the route of BHO, make sure the material is tested for residual solvents. No one wants to be inhaling butane.

CO_2 Oil. This concentrate commonly preloaded in vape pens is made from an extraction using CO_2, considered one of the safest solvents for industrial extraction.

Distillate. Ultra-refined cannabis concentrates from butane or CO_2 extractions, further distilled down to extremely high THC concentrations without the benefit of other cannabinoids or terpenes.

Hash. Soft and pliant plant material, made from concentrated kief. Hardens with time and with exposure to air.

Kief. Powdery plant material from plant resin.

Resin. While resin is what the plant naturally produces, "resin" you see in shops will likely refer to a concentrate made with butane. The distinction of "Live Resin" will indicate that the concentrate was made when the plant was freshly harvested, thus retaining the greatest amount of terpenes.

Rosin. A solventless concentrate made by pressing and heating the material to excrete the resin and separate it from the more fibrous parts of the plant. The term "Live Rosin" will indicate that the plant material was freshly harvested, and since it's still a solventless process, this is a pretty unbeatable option in terms of taste, effect, and health benefits.

Shatter. Typically a clear sheet of highly concentrated material, produced by the extraction with solvents.

Wax/Crumble. Crumbly, sticky, and waxy bits of concentrate. Generic term for various processes that produce a sticky, concentrated form of THC.

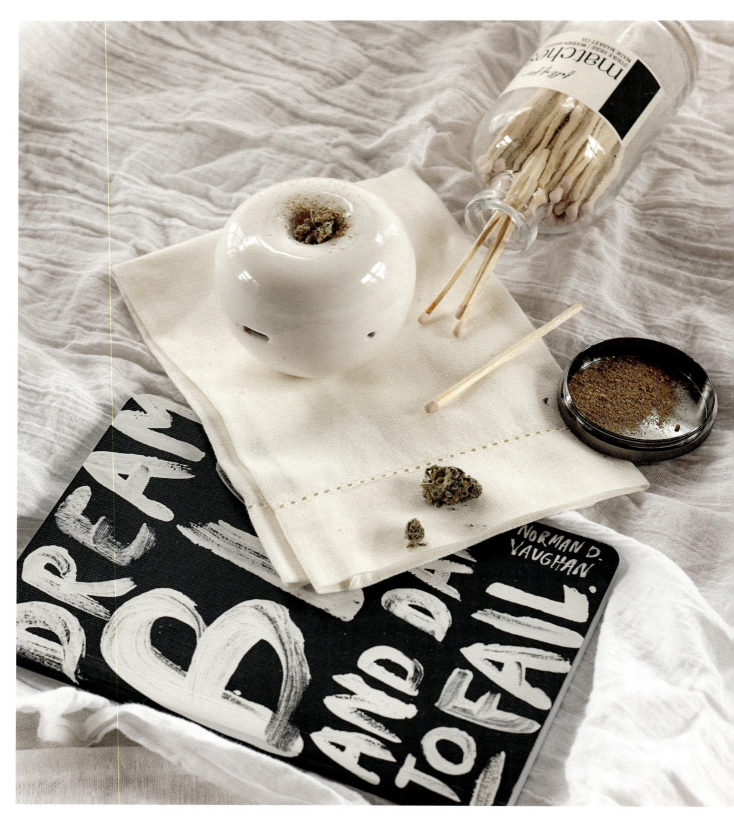

Finding Your Dose

Everyone reacts to the different strains of cannabis and their various delivery methods in different ways. I cannot stress enough that finding your comfortable cannabis potency is key to a pleasant and healthy experience. It is easy to overdo it, so take the time to find the right product, dose, and delivery method for you.

Start with 2.5 to 5 milligrams of THC for ingestibles and wait at least four hours before having more. If inhaling, have a couple of puffs and wait fifteen minutes before increasing your dose. Every time you medicate with cannabis, your reaction might be a bit different. The strain and strength of the cannabis might play into it, just like what you've had to eat recently might. The only reliable way to achieve the same effects would be to have the same strain from the same grower's batch or the same product under the same conditions. It is important to keep a record of what works and what doesn't—and why. Use a scale from 1 to 10 to explain the intensity of your high, 1 being no high and 10 being way too high. Keep a log of your cannabis use to find the right dose and delivery method for you. There are cannabis journals on the market that can assist you in your journey. We recommend the cannabis journal from Goldleaf.

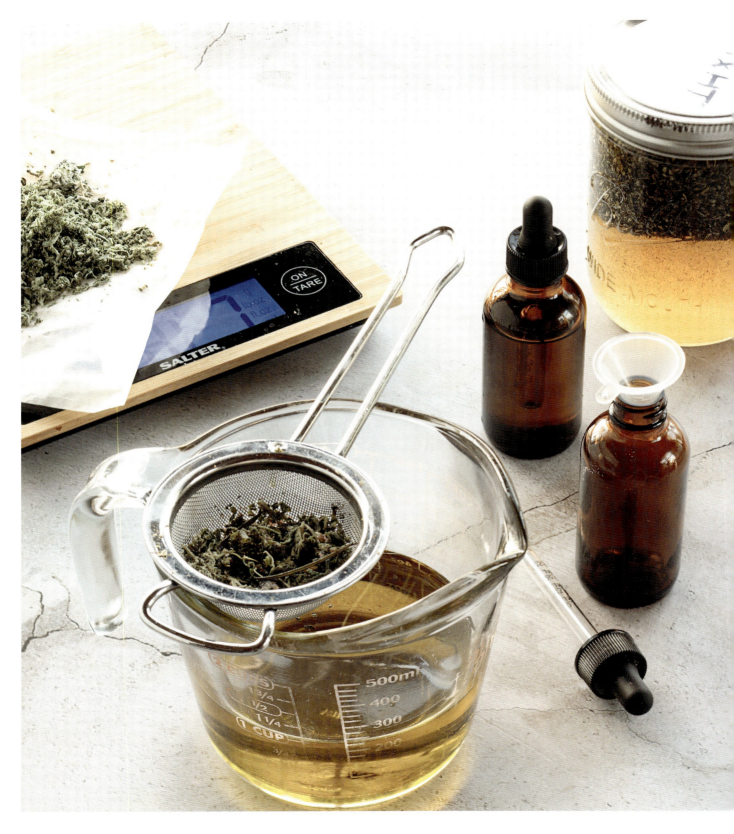

How to Make a Basic Tincture
Using THC or CBD

Yield: 12 ounces | Serving: 2.5 milliliters / 50 drops / ¹/₂ teaspoon per serving
THC/CBD: 5 milligrams per serving (720 milligrams total)

While many tinctures are alcohol-based, we opt for the gentleness and sweet taste of tinctures made with vegetable glycerin. Like oil infusions, this glycerin tincture will become saturated with the cannabinoids and terpenes from your cannabis or hemp. This allows you to customize your tincture to fit your needs and requirements.

THC

7 grams cannabis, coarsely ground

12 ounces vegetable glycerin

To make a THC tincture, we used cannabis with 15 percent THC for a resulting serving size of about 5 milligrams THC per ¹/₂ teaspoon. You may want to use more or less cannabis depending on your preferred dosage level.

CBD

7 grams hemp, coarsely ground

12 ounces vegetable glycerin

To make a CBD tincture, we used hemp with 15 percent CBD for a resulting serving size of about 5 milligrams CBD per ¹/₂ teaspoon. You may want to use more or less hemp depending on your preferred dosage level.

THC & CBD

7 grams cannabis, coarsely ground

7 grams hemp, coarsely ground

12 ounces vegetable glycerin

To make a tincture with both THC and CBD, you can either use a cannabis strain with both cannabinoids or use both cannabis and hemp in your process. We used hemp with 15 percent CBD and cannabis with 15 percent THC for a resulting serving size of about 5 milligrams CBD and 5 milligrams THC per ¹/₂ teaspoon. Again, you may want to use more or less depending on your preferred dosage level.

1. Place the cannabis and/or hemp in a turkey roasting bag (optional) on a baking sheet in a 240°F/116°C oven for 45 minutes to activate the THC and/or CBD (decarboxylate).

2. Transfer the decarboxylated cannabis and/or hemp to a clean glass jar.

3. Pour the glycerin into the jar, being sure that the glycerin covers the cannabis and/or hemp completely.

4. Secure the jar with an airtight lid and gently mix the contents by rolling the jar back and forth in your hands.

5. Keep the jar in a dark place near room temperature for about 2 months. Gently shake the jar every few days.

6. After 2 months, strain the plant material from the tincture. Stretch cheesecloth across the top of a large spouted measuring cup or bowl and secure with a rubber band or twine around the edge.

7. Carefully pour the infused glycerin over the cheesecloth.

8. Lift the cheesecloth and squeeze any remaining glycerin into the measuring cup or bowl. Discard the cheesecloth and solids.

9. Pour the glycerin back into the glass jar or into dropper bottles if you have them. Keep in a cool, dark place.

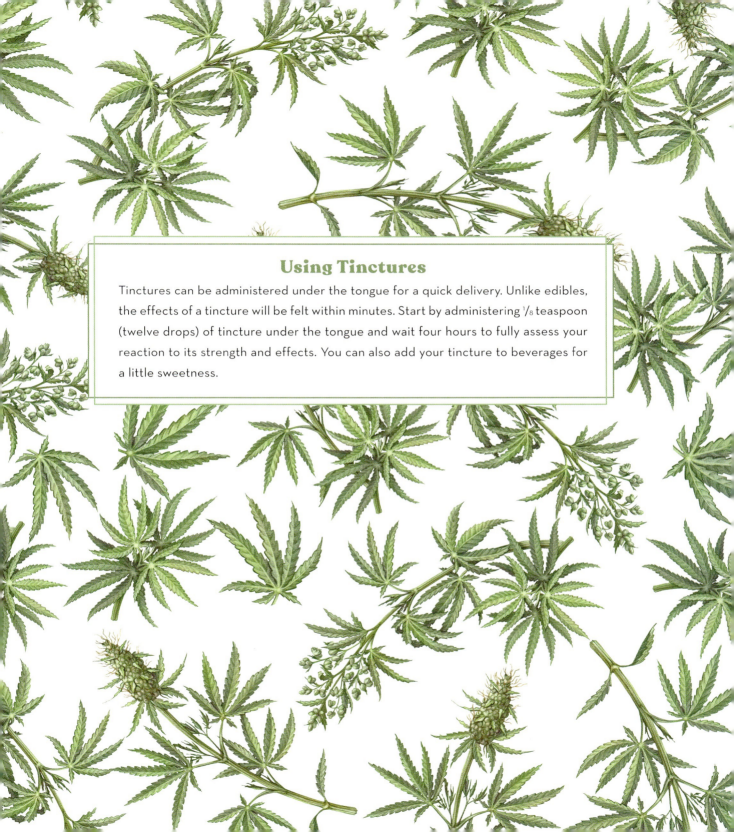

Using Tinctures

Tinctures can be administered under the tongue for a quick delivery. Unlike edibles, the effects of a tincture will be felt within minutes. Start by administering $\frac{1}{8}$ teaspoon (twelve drops) of tincture under the tongue and wait four hours to fully assess your reaction to its strength and effects. You can also add your tincture to beverages for a little sweetness.

How to Make Capsules Using THC or CBD

Yield: 200 capsules | Serving: 1 capsule | THC/CBD: 5 milligrams per serving

Capsules are a great way to ingest a consistent amount of cannabis easily and efficiently. To make your own capsules, you will need a capsule machine and empty size OO capsules. To administer, start with 1 capsule and wait 4 hours to fully assess your reaction to its strength and effects.

THC

9 grams cannabis, coarsely ground

7 ounces coconut oil

To make a THC capsule, we used cannabis with 15 percent THC for a resulting dosage of 5 milligrams each. You may want to use more or less cannabis depending on your dosage level.

CBD

9 grams hemp, coarsely ground

7 ounces coconut oil

To make a CBD capsule, we used hemp with 15 percent THC for a resulting dosage of 5 milligrams each. You may want to use more or less hemp depending on your dosage level.

THC & CBD

9 grams cannabis, coarsely ground

9 grams hemp, coarsely ground

7 ounces coconut oil

To make a THC & CBD capsule, you can either use a cannabis strain with both cannabinoids or use both cannabis and hemp in your process. We used cannabis with 15 percent THC and a hemp strain with 15 percent CBD for a resulting dosage of 5 milligrams THC and 5 milligrams CBD each. You may want to use more or less cannabis, depending on your dosage level.

1. Place the cannabis and/or hemp on a rimmed baking sheet in a 240°F/116°C oven for 45 minutes to activate the THC and/or CBD (decarboxylate).

2. Heat the coconut oil in a small saucepan over low heat. Add the decarboxylated cannabis to the oil. Stir to mix.

3. Cook for 3 hours over very low heat, stirring occasionally. The oil should not boil or simmer, although occasional bubbles are okay.

4. Line a fine mesh strainer with cheesecloth and place it over a large heat-safe bowl.

5. Carefully pour the oil through the cheesecloth and allow the excess oil to drain through.

6. Once the mixture has cooled just enough to handle, lift the cheesecloth and squeeze any remaining oil into the bowl.

7. Follow the instructions from the capsule machine to make the capsules. You may need a tapered syringe to help fill all the capsules. Fill while the coconut oil is still in liquid form. If it solidifies before you fill the capsules, reheat it on the stove over low heat.

8. Store the capsules in an airtight container in the refrigerator.

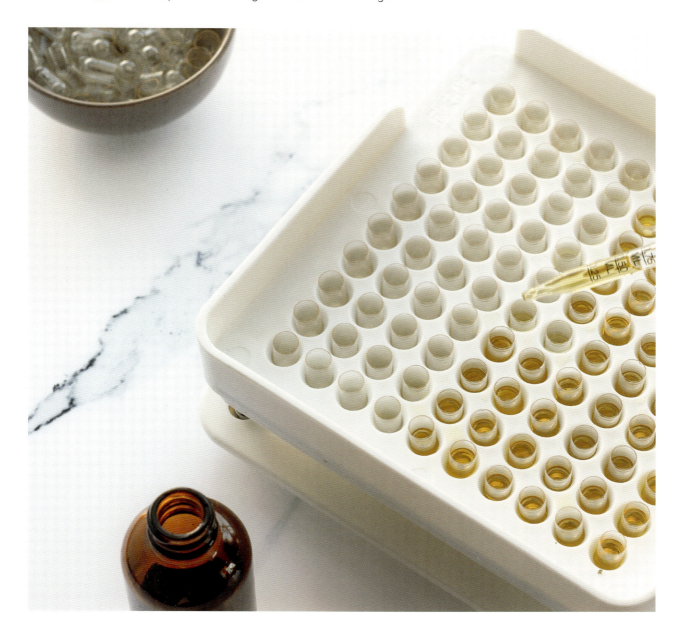

Finding Quality Cannabis

When you enter a dispensary for the first time, you are likely to be blown away. The variety of flower, as well as all the different cannabis products, all in one place, can be a little mind-boggling. I remarked after my first dispensary experience that I felt the way Imelda Marcos would have felt walking into Jimmy Choo's. There are flowers (buds), concentrates, edibles, topicals, and tinctures—and subcategories within these categories! Don't be afraid to ask questions until you have an understanding of the options, their uses, and their effects.

If you are a cannabis newbie, this can all feel both a little exciting and a little terrifying. If you follow the directions of your budtender (and doctor), you should have a very pleasant and interesting experience.

Step one is to find a dispensary. You can refer to weedmaps.com or leafly.com to find the dispensaries closest to you. These websites also have menus of the shop's offerings (the strains in their menu may even have cannabinoid and terpenes profiles—a helpful research tool!) and reviews from patients, just like Yelp. This is a great place to start your dispensary search, but nothing beats a face-to-face discussion with one of the dispensary's budtenders—or budistas, as I like to call them.

Knowledgeable, caring staff can make all the difference. Budistas at a reputable dispensary will know their stuff and be able to work with you to find what you are looking for. If you do not feel comfortable in a specific dispensary, don't hesitate to move on to the next place until you find the right match. Dispensaries have different vibes and cater to different audiences. Look around and find a good fit.

The next step after you've found a dispensary that you like is choosing what cannabis to buy, which can be a challenge. With hundreds of strains available, how will you know which strain is right for you? Your goal is to find a strain of cannabis that will give you the effects and relief that you need. In order to meet this goal, there are certain things you will need to watch out for and avoid. Ask the budtender about testing requirements for cannabis and be sure you only purchase products that have tested negative for pesticides, contaminants, mold, and mildew. These are nasty chemicals to inhale or ingest and are to be avoided.

With the help of your budtender, you can and should find out the name of the farm that grew the cannabis, when the cannabis was harvested, whether the cannabis is pesticide free, and the potency of the strain. In most dispensaries, the potency of cannabis flower and various extracts will be expressed as a percentage of the item's overall weight. The THC content of buds tends to be in the 20 to 30 percent range around Oregon, while extracts are in the 50 to 80 percent range. When you're shopping, you should look for these percentages, as well as for the percentages of other cannabinoids, to get a full picture of the plant's profile. (See Chapter 2 for an overview of the cannabinoids to look for.)

A good budtender will be able to work with you to get the cannabis effects you desire. Before you go to your chosen dispensary, it's worth spending some time making a list of the effects you're hoping to achieve, as well as any particular effects you might be hoping to avoid. For instance, if you have considerable anxiety you should be sure to mention that. Some strains can actually increase anxiety. If you have trouble sleeping, that should also factor in to what strain you buy. There are strains that will keep you up and wired, which some people like and others don't. If you have pain, be sure to share that info as well. Having any recent medical test results available when you go to buy a new strain is a game changer.

When shopping for cannabis, your nose will be a huge help. A strong aroma, be it pungent, citrusy, or earthy, is a good sign. Look for buds that are vibrant and colorful. You want your flower to range in color from deep green with orange hairs to purple or blue. Pass on dry brown buds; you will be disappointed. High-quality cannabis will feel sticky and resinous, not dry or crumbly.

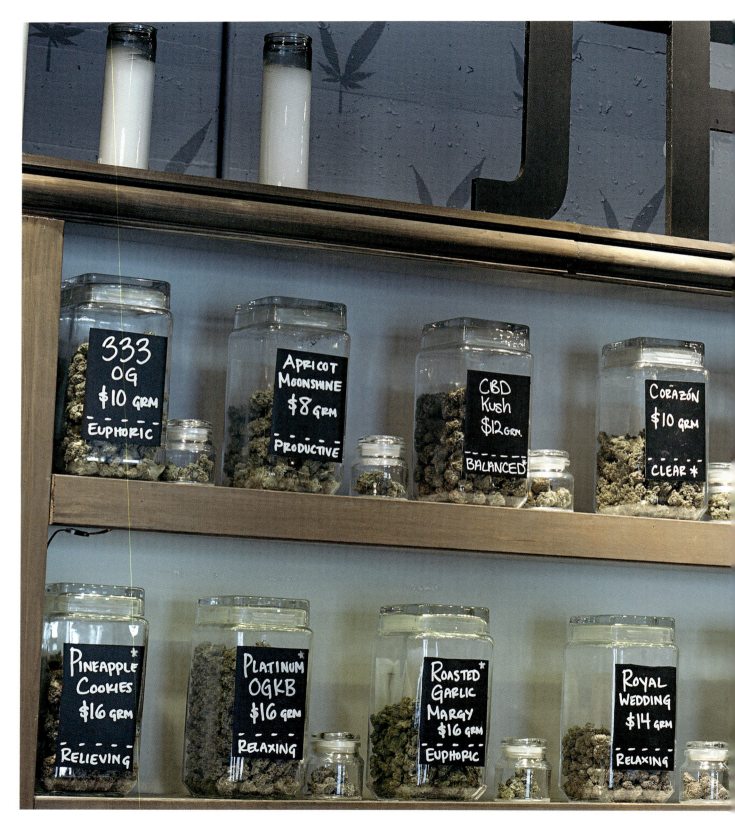

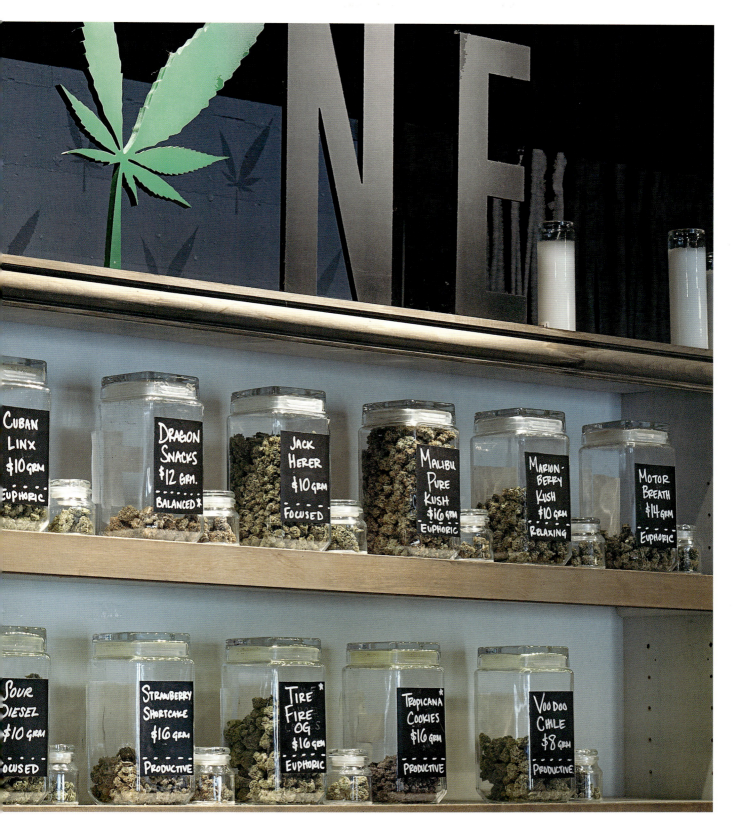

Responsible Use and Consumption

It's pretty simple. Cannabis is safe when used responsibly and under the proper conditions. Remember that cannabis with THC will alter your thinking, reflexes, mobility, and ability to use restraint when around food!

Here are some rules to follow. Be a champ and respect the plant.

- Don't drive
- Don't give cannabis to children
- Don't be irresponsible
- Be careful when mixing alcohol and cannabis; proceed with caution

- Pick a safe place to ingest
- Be with people you trust
- Don't go overboard

What to Do If You've Had Too Much

Consuming too much cannabis, in any form, is a rather unpleasant experience. You may feel dizzy and confused, possibly nauseated, anxious, and paranoid. No fun at all. You won't die, but you will count the seconds till it wears off. For me, getting in bed, lying still, and maybe listening to music is my go-to way of coping with overindulgence. The worst of it is usually over in less than an hour, but that hour can feel like a lifetime. If you have a high CBD strain on hand, you should consume a small dose, as it will help inhibit the psychoactive effects of THC.

Even if you don't have any CBD on hand, you can still make sure to stay hydrated, and it's always a good idea to distract yourself by watching a sweet movie that is pure fun. *Ratatouille* is my favorite movie to watch while under the influence.

Some folks say that black peppercorns may help, and others laud the effects of citrus drinks. Whatever method you have for dealing with overindulgence, the larger lesson is simple: When it comes to cannabis, less is more. When you feel like you've reached a comfortable place, stop. Too much cannabis is not a good thing.

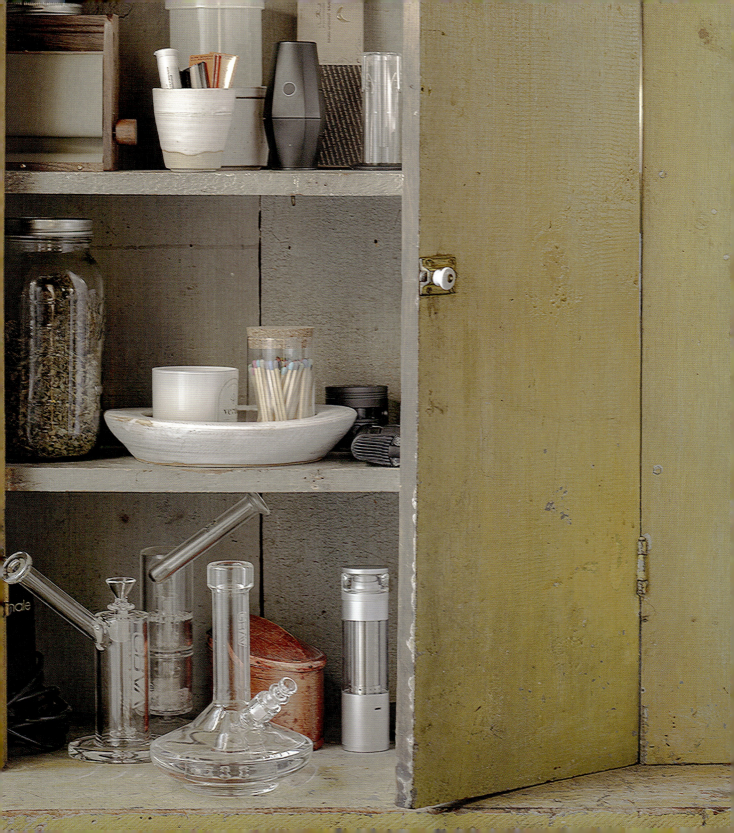

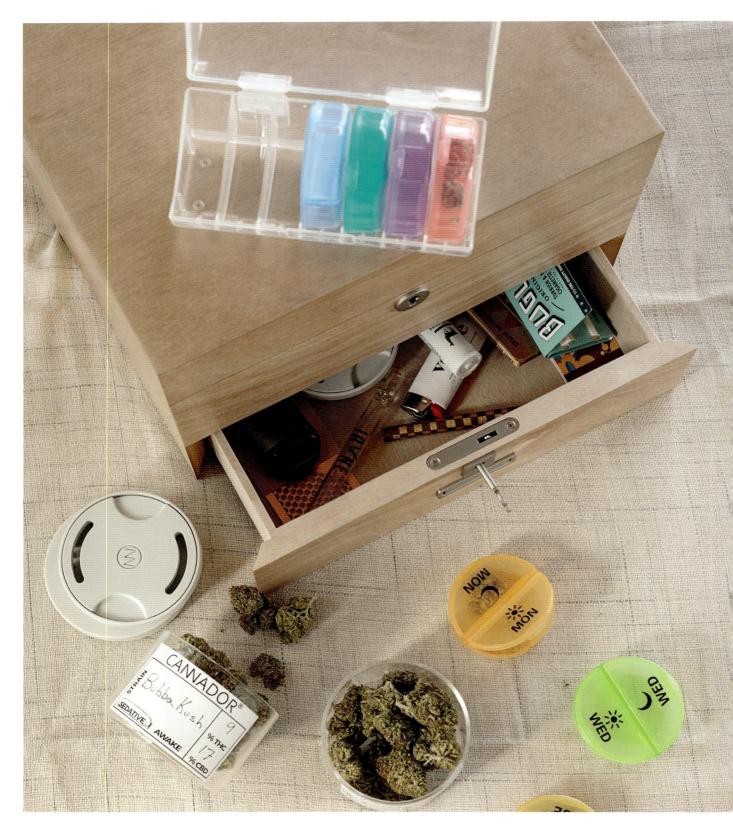

Storing Cannabis

Light and heat are the greatest threats to the flower, as the same UV rays that we protect ourselves from with sunscreen and clothing will damage the important cannabinoids and terpenes in the plant. Air is another issue for storage—too much can cause the cannabis to degrade.

There are some pretty cool products out there that are perfect for keeping your cannabis in mint condition. When choosing a storage container, make sure that it is the correct size. Stuffing cannabis into a jar or bag that's too small may damage the flower, causing you to crush the buds and possibly even lose precious bits of resinous kief. If the container is too big, excess air will potentially degrade the plant. A vacuum sealer, if you happen to have one, will take care of your surplus air issues.

Another potential issue with cannabis storage is moisture. Moisture can cause mold, which will absolutely ruin your cannabis. Make sure that your cannabis is dry but not too dry. Proper humidity is key to successful storage. There are humidity control packets (Boveda is the one we use), and they really seem to do the trick.

Finally, keep your stored cannabis in a temperature-stable environment. High temperatures will cause the flower to dry out and degrade, and you may lose valuable terpenes.

In recent years, there have been a few weed humidors made available, though they cost several hundred dollars. They will maintain a steady temperature, humidity, and protection from light.

Growing Cannabis at Home: Steps to Full Plant

If you live in a state that allows for growing cannabis at home, this is your lucky day/ year. Growing cannabis, inside or outside, will allow you to pick the strain that works best for you. You can start with seeds or a clone/cutting from a plant.

Growing your own cannabis is relaxing and fun, and it can save you money. For a step-by-step guide, *The Cannabis Grow Bible* by Greg Green is a wonderful resource. If you have a friend who grows, it's always nice to get personalized help.

If you can, start growing with a clone, a cutting from a "mother" cannabis plant. They are often available in dispensaries, hopefully with strain information, including terpenes and cannabinoids. If you can't get a clone, there are hundreds of seeds available online, with all the strain information you might want.

Once your crop begins to grow, you should make sure to remove male plants that develop, unless you are interested in growing seeds. Unlike most plants that flower, cannabis needs a male and a female plant to reproduce. Male plants must be removed or the female plants will start producing seeds rather than the big beautiful buds you are looking for. To identify the sex of the plant before it enters its flower stage, you'll have to take a peek between its nodes. At about six weeks, the plant will enter a pre-flowering stage where it produces hairlike calyxes or ball-like pollen sacs. If it's balls, it's a male; throw it out. But do so carefully to make sure you don't shake any pollen onto nearby females.

Choose a large container for your plant. There are some great pots that are inexpensive and will allow your plant to thrive. Grow your cannabis in a room that will maintain a temperature between 65 and 80 degrees Fahrenheit (18 to 27 degrees Celsius) with twelve hours of sunlight. If you live in a climate that meets these conditions, you can grow outside. Otherwise you need to set up an indoor grow. In this case, you need to set up a small, well-ventilated area and mount an LED grow

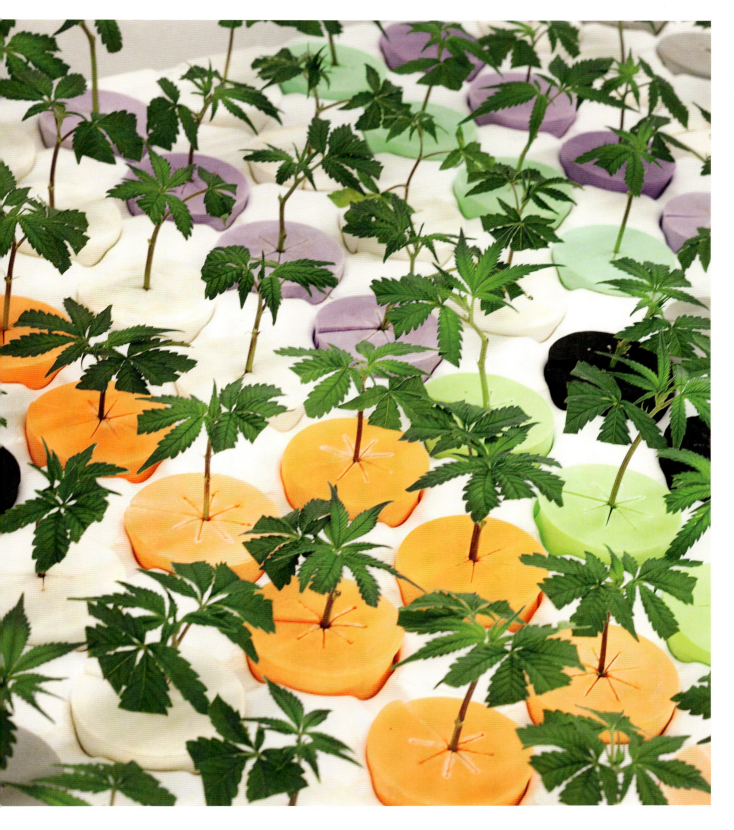

light above your plant. You should also set up a small fan to keep the air moving. During the first four weeks of indoor growing, you should light your plant for eighteen hours a day, then give it six hours of rest in the dark. After the first four weeks, you can switch to a twelve-hours-on, twelve-hours-off schedule, which will help initiate the flowering stage. From this point, it will be another two to three months before your plant is ready. Using a magnifying glass, look at the buds' resinous trichomes. The plants are ready to harvest when the trichomes begin to turn from clear to amber and milky.

You will know to harvest when the plants tell you they are ready. When the pistils (the hairlike parts on the bud) darken and begin to curl, it's time. Cut off all the branches, remove the fan leaves, trim the large sugar leaves (leaves close to the buds that are covered in some amount of resin), and hang them upside down to dry or use a mesh drying rack. Let the leaves dry uncovered for a week. Next, place the buds in closed glass jars and cure for two weeks. Open the jars at least once a day for the first two weeks and then every couple of days if you want to continue the curing process for a longer period of time. Two weeks will do the trick, but some people cure their leaves for up to six months. Like a fine wine, some believe that giving a cannabis leaf more time to age improves its quality.

After the curing process is complete, your cannabis is officially ready for action.

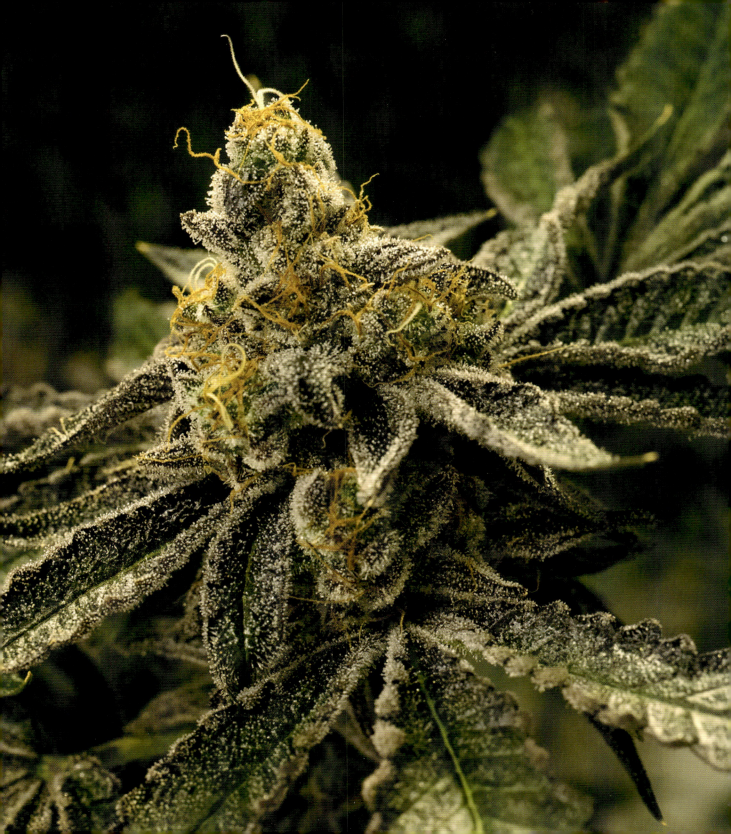

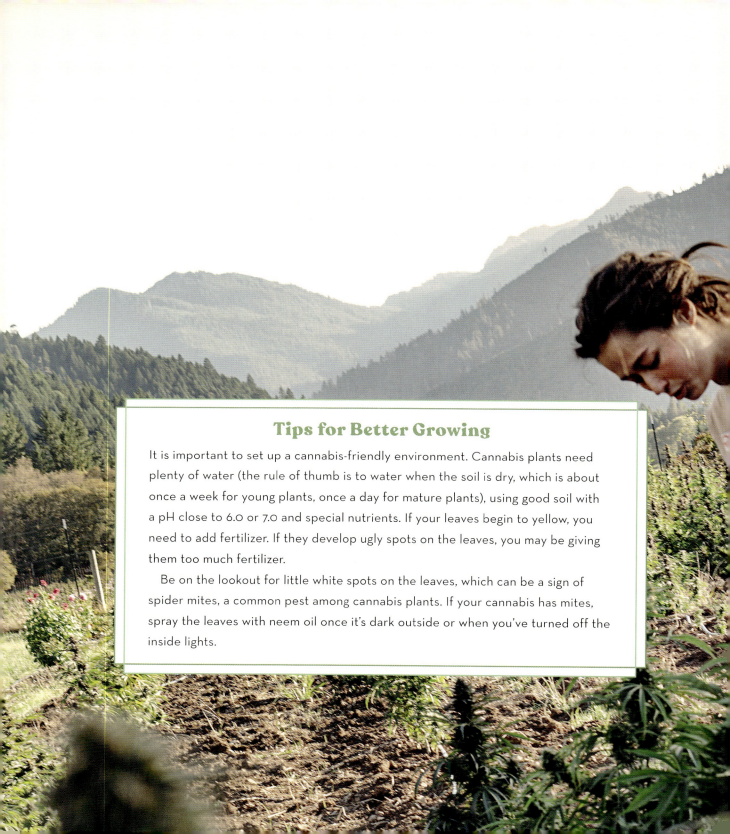

Tips for Better Growing

It is important to set up a cannabis-friendly environment. Cannabis plants need plenty of water (the rule of thumb is to water when the soil is dry, which is about once a week for young plants, once a day for mature plants), using good soil with a pH close to 6.0 or 7.0 and special nutrients. If your leaves begin to yellow, you need to add fertilizer. If they develop ugly spots on the leaves, you may be giving them too much fertilizer.

Be on the lookout for little white spots on the leaves, which can be a sign of spider mites, a common pest among cannabis plants. If your cannabis has mites, spray the leaves with neem oil once it's dark outside or when you've turned off the inside lights.

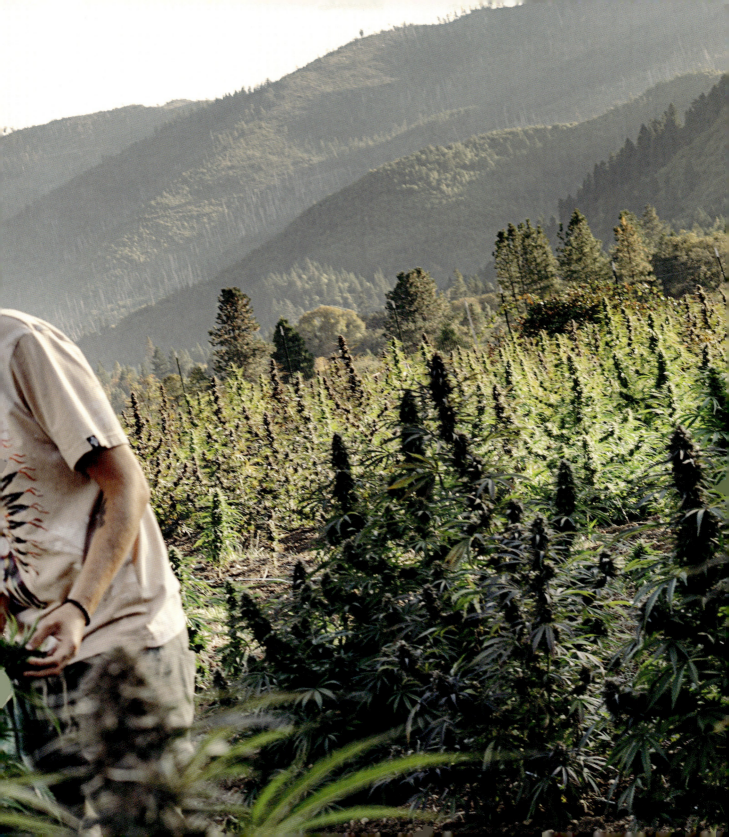

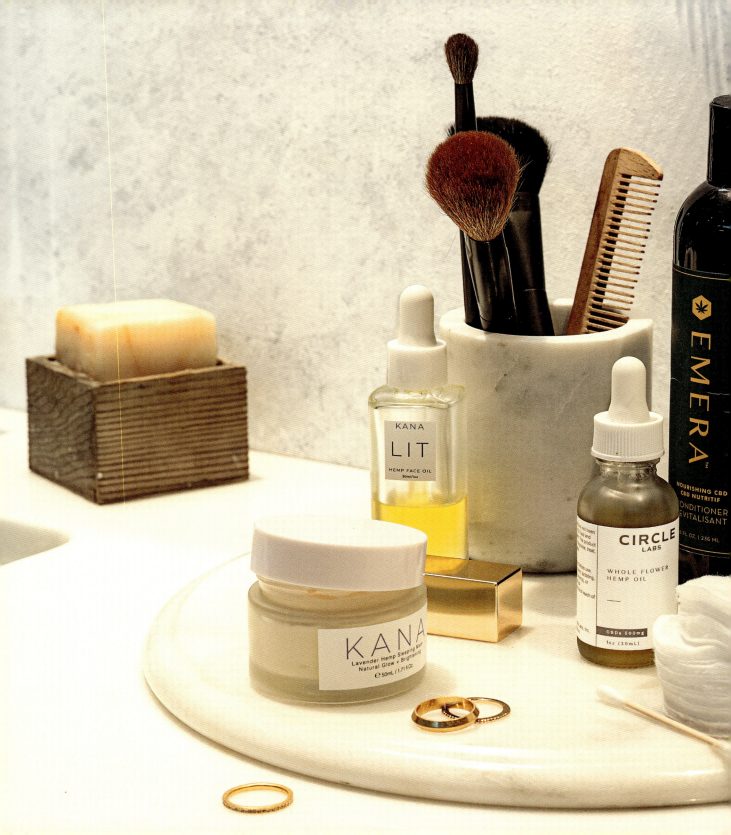

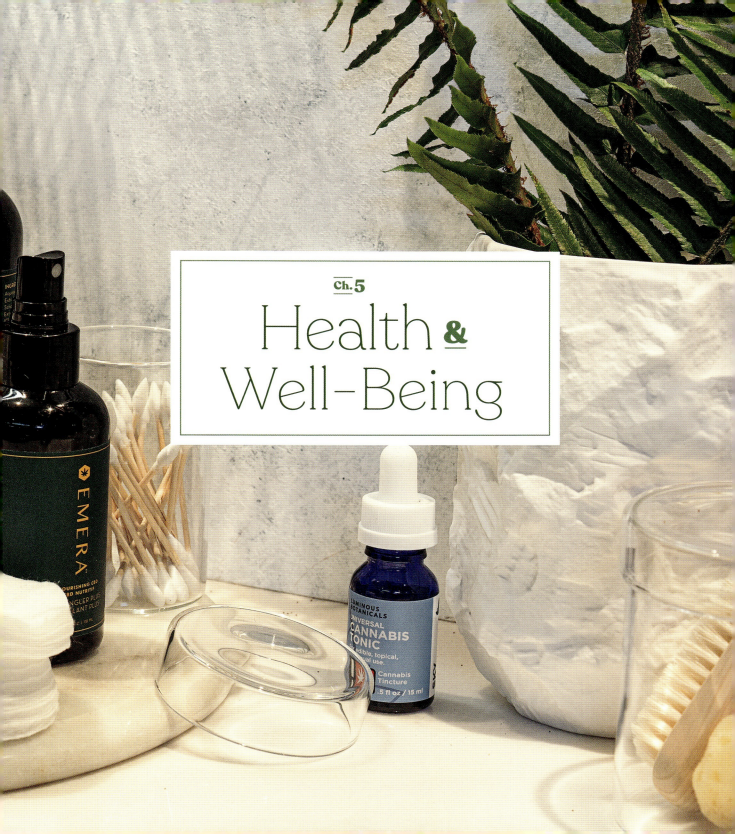

Ch. 5

Health & Well-Being

As the use of cannabis becomes more prevalent both in the United States and around the world, the range of cannabis-based products continues to grow. Many of these items are available without a prescription, and there's a product for nearly every body part. Seriously. There is a stunning array of products on the market to help users manage various health issues, ranging from lack of sleep to nausea associated with chemotherapy. I manage my seizure disorder with cannabis, which has allowed me to stop using prescription meds that have serious side effects. And I've got to say, cannabis lube is pretty spectacular. Mary and I once attended a cannabis event—this was back in the day when there was a ton of weed given out and enjoyed—and I mixed up samples and drank the lube. No, it was not a *Deep Throat* moment, just another story from this crazy cannabis journey we are on.

Cannabis for Sleep

As mentioned in Chapter 3, cannabis can be an excellent therapy for insomnia and other sleep disorders. But you'll likely need to experiment. While some people find it relaxing to consume cannabis before bed, saying it helps them drift effortlessly to sleep, for others, it can make the mind and heart race. It all depends on your unique endocannabinoid system, your sensitivity to THC, and the specific cultivar you use.

If you're using cannabis as a sleep aid, seek out strains that are rich in terpenes like myrcene or linalool, both of which have sedating effects. If you're sensitive to THC, you may also want to try CBD by itself, since it has been shown to reduce anxiety, which can often lead to sleeplessness. Others find the perfect combination for sleep is a 2:1 ratio of CBD to THC—whether in the form of cannabis flower, a tincture, or an edible. You may also want to experiment with what time you take cannabis prior to sleep. Try keeping a cannabis sleep journal. Goldleaf makes a beautiful Patient Journal for tracking the effect cannabis has on different maladies.

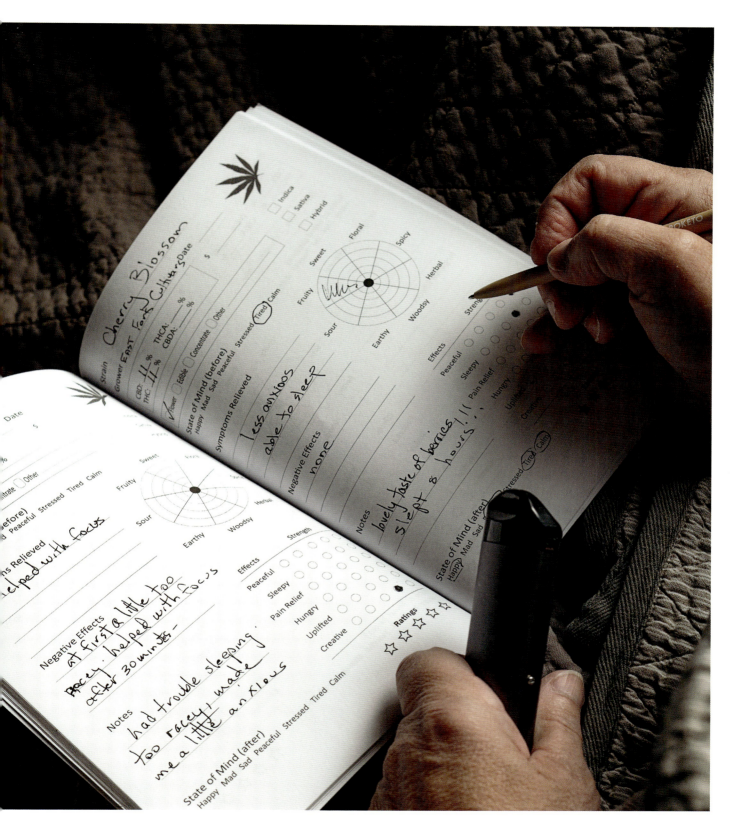

Right page

Strain **Cherry Blossom**

Grower **EAST Fork Cultivars** Date

$

☐ Indica
☐ Sativa
☐ Hybrid

CBD: **11** % THCA: _____ %
THC: **11** % CBDA: _____ %

☑ Flower ☐ Edible ☐ Concentrate ☐ Other

State of Mind (before)
Happy Mad Sad Peaceful Stressed (Tired) Calm

Symptoms Relieved
less anxious
able to sleep

Negative Effects
none

(aroma wheel: Floral, Spicy, Sweet, Herbal, Fruity, Woodsy, Sour, Earthy)

Strength

Effects
Peaceful
Sleepy
Pain Relief
Hungry
Uplifted
Creative

Notes lovely taste of berries!!!
slept 8 hours...

State of Mind (after)
Happy Mad Sad Peaceful (Stressed) (Tired) (Calm)

Left page

Date

$

% itrate ☐ Other

before)
d Peaceful Stressed Tired Calm

ns Relieved
lped with focus

(aroma wheel: Sweet, Fruity, Sour, Earthy, Woodsy, Herbal)

Strength

Effects
Peaceful
Sleepy
Pain Relief
Hungry
Uplifted
Creative

Ratings ☆ ☆ ☆
☆ ☆ ☆ ☆

Negative Effects
at first a little too
racey. helped with focus
after 30 minutes -

Notes had trouble sleeping.
too racey. made
me a little anxious

State of Mind (after)
Happy Mad Sad Peaceful Stressed Tired Calm

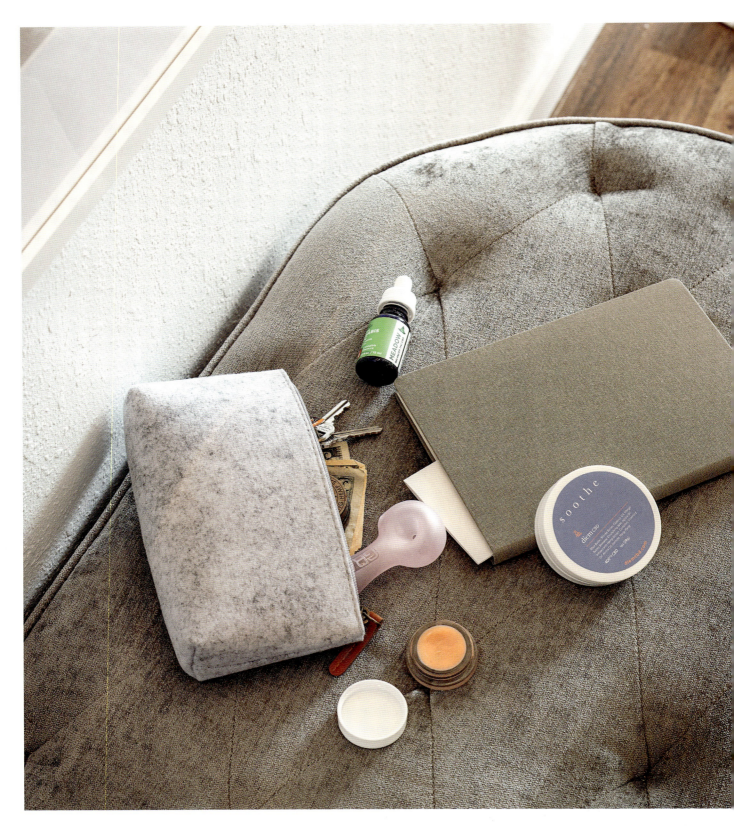

There are a growing number of products on the market these days using hemp and cannabis to promote uninterrupted sleep. You can use cannabis indirectly to help you get a better night's sleep by taking a bubble bath with a cannabis bath bomb (Kush Queen makes one specifically for restful sleep), applying Kana Skincare's lavender hemp sleeping mask, and rubbing Dr. Kerklaan's Natural Sleep Cream (with CBD and melatonin as well as citrus and lavender) all over your neck and shoulders. You'll be drifting off to sleep, flying through fields of luscious hemp, in no time.

Topicals for Pain Relief

Since it's well-established that cannabis works for pain, using topicals is a no-brainer (and no, they won't get you high!). In every state that has legalized cannabis, balms, lotions, and relief oils—often combining cannabis with aromatherapeutic elements like arnica, lavender, and menthol—are flying off the shelves. That's because, quite simply, they work. People use them for arthritis pain, sore muscles, sprains and strains, and even neuropathy. You just want to be sure that the product you buy has been tested and clearly lists the potency of THC and other cannabinoids it may contain. Aim for 4.5 milligrams of cannabinoids per gram (0.45 percent) of product. So, for example, a 28-gram container of salve should contain around 120 milligrams of THC.

Rescue Rub, made by Peak Extracts in Portland, Oregon, makes topicals for pain and inflammation. The salve, made with a lightweight base of coconut, shea, and jojoba oils, comes in two versions: One is made with 0.43 percent THC and twelve herbs, including angelica, bergamot, and rose; the other is a 2:1 ratio of CBD to THC, and the same blend of herbs. Susan Vaughan, a high school teacher from St. Paul, Minnesota, was sure her knee injury would keep her from participating in the Oregon half marathon she'd signed up for six months earlier. At the urging of a friend, she slathered some Peak Extracts (the THC-only kind) on her knee twice in the day before the race. Her knee pain dissipated, and she was able to endure all thirteen miles. "The tightness in my knee was still there, but I was able to do the entire race without pain," says Vaughan. She was even able to run around three of the thirteen miles. "That's amazing, considering I had not run in a long time."

Emerging research is showing that THCA can regulate inflammation and pain sensations in the skin. Trista Okel, founder and CEO of Portland's Empower BodyCare, is a THCA believer. All of her THC-infused products, including her Topical Relief Oil, contain THCA and CBD in a 1:1 ratio, with a little bit of THC to "open up" the CB1 receptors of the skin. CBD does not directly interact with CB1 receptors, but it does activate receptors that regulate pain, temperature, and inflammation. Once again, the synergistic combination of cannabinoids seems to be more effective than when they're used individually.

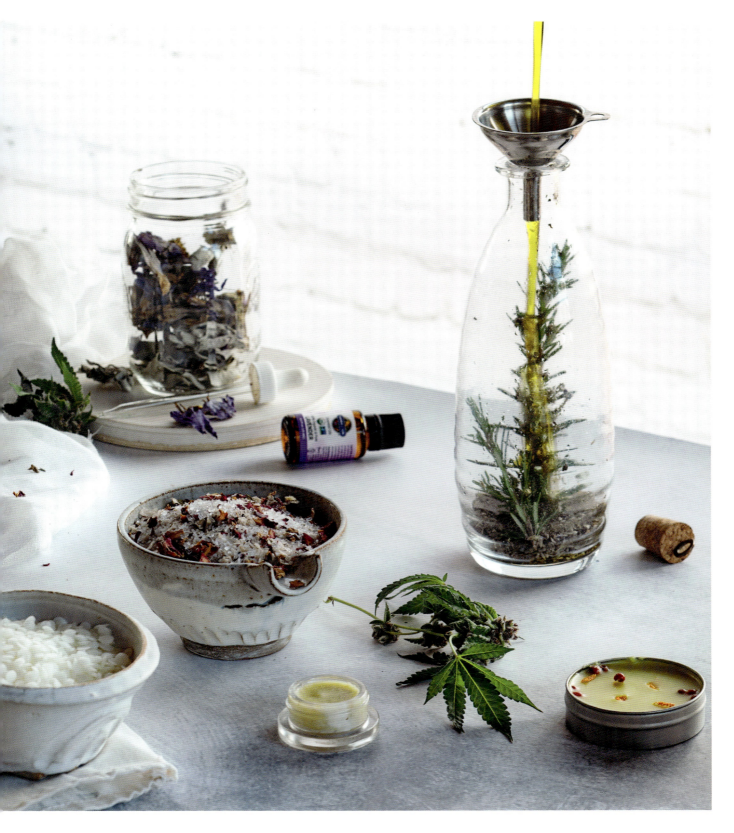

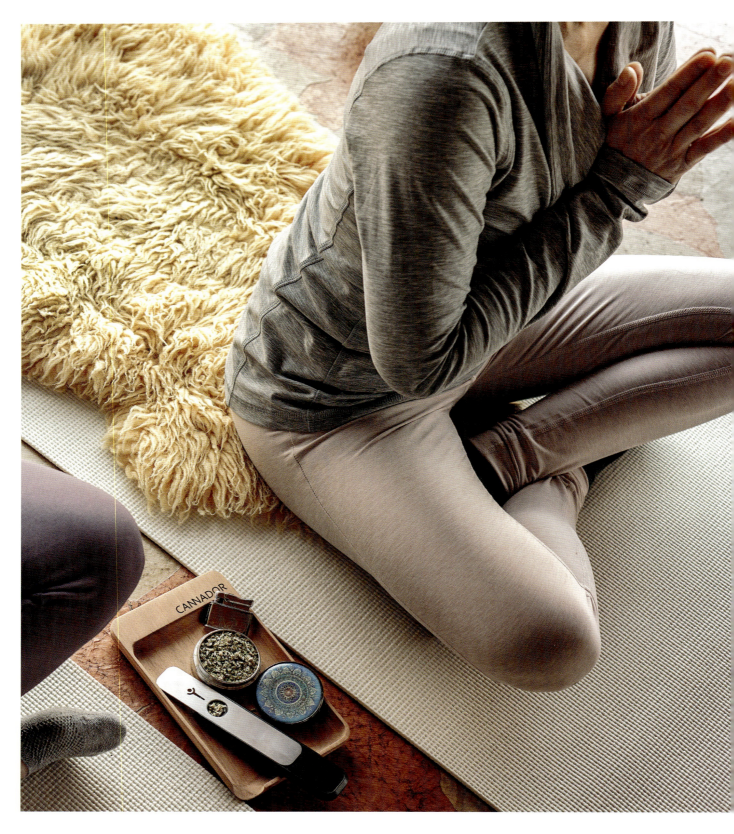

Cannabis and Yoga

People have been smoking weed and going to yoga classes stoned for years. But now, with so many states legalizing cannabis, weed-infused yoga classes are openly advertised. There's Higher Self Yoga in Los Angeles, a ganja yoga class at Denver's cannabis co-working space Cultivated Synergy, Stoned Yoga at Jayne dispensary in Portland, Oregon, the Local Yoga Joint in western Massachusetts, and many more.

Yoga teacher and cannabis enthusiast Jocelyn O'Shea founded Local Yoga Joint in Turners Falls, Massachusetts, because she wanted to create a safe space for people to openly smoke weed and do yoga. "Finally, the laws have changed and we're able to do this," O'Shea says. Cannabis, she continues, allows you to be super present and explore the internal world: "As much as it's interesting to get stoned and watch the trees move around, when you look inward, there's a whole mass of things going on. It kind of opens the door in a different way." In addition to consumption-friendly classes, her studio hosts educational workshops on CBD, edibles and yoga, and cannabis basics. For those who are still wary of getting high, she offers a few CBD-infused restorative classes. "We start out with a piece of CBD chocolate—you let it melt in your mouth during a guided meditation," she says. Then, between each posture, she instructs students to either use a CBD salve or tincture before relaxing into the next posture. "It's awesome. After those classes, everyone feels so good! Really clear and relaxed," O'Shea says.

In Portland, there's even a cannabis-centric fitness experience called Mary Jane Fonda that combines an aerobic workout with yoga. Founder Amarett Jans launched Mary Jane Fonda after Donald Trump was elected as a way to bring people together. "I knew there was going to be a community of people that needed a release—and a place to be themselves," she says. "It just seemed like, with that bad news of the president, this would be an outlet." She incorporated aerobics because she was interested in "a bit more sparkle" than yoga could provide.

Bath Soaks

Soaking in a hot bath is already an established remedy for relaxing, soothing sore muscles, and letting go of all your cares. What better way to incorporate cannabis into your life than by adding it to your bathtub? It's no wonder that bath bombs and bath salts—either made with CBD only or with a combination of CBD and THC—have become hugely popular from coast to coast.

In California, Kush Queen has a handful of popular bath bombs, each of which contains CBD alone, or CBD and THC together (25 milligrams of each). Relieve, with a blend of clove, birch, rosemary, black pepper, and coriander, is for pain and sore muscles. Sleep, which contains lavender, mandarin orange, and marjoram, provides intense relaxation and calm. And Awaken energizes with a blend of peppermint oil. There are nine other kinds of bath bombs, and some limited-edition ones as well. As usual, you can order the CBD-only bath bombs online, but the ones containing THC have to be purchased at a licensed dispensary.

San Francisco–based Jamie Evans, founder of the cannabis blog and lifestyle brand the Herb Somm, loves Om Edibles' cannabis-infused Epsom bath salts. "I use the lavender one on a daily basis," says Evans. There are four others: rose geranium; athletic (made with a therapeutic level of essential oils); lemon, ginger, and eucalyptus; and fragrance free. All contain 25 milligrams each of THC and CBD. She's also a fan of Papa & Barkley's Releaf Soak, with eucalyptus, tea tree, peppermint, and lavender (and a 3:1 ratio of THC to CBD). "It's the perfect remedy for after sports," says Evans.

Oregon's Empower BodyCare makes two kinds of bath salts. One is CBD-infused, mixed with lavender and bergamot. The other, available only at licensed dispensaries in Oregon and Washington, contains equal parts CBD and THCA (with a tiny bit of THC), as well as lavender and bergamot. Both are great ways to relax and de-stress, but the latter is a more potent combination for sore muscles and pain.

Rose Bath Salts

Yield: 16 ounces | Serving: 4 ounces per bath

A long, hot bath is one of my very favorite things. I'll put on a good album, light up a joint, and enjoy an hour of pure bliss. Adding CBD and THC to bath salts elevates the experience and produces a head-to-toe feeling of relaxation unlike any other.

1 cup Epsom salt

1 cup coarse sea salt

1 tablespoon infused coconut oil

5 drops peppermint essential oil

5 drops sweet orange essential oil

10 drops rosemary essential oil

Dried rose petals

1. Mix the Epsom salt and sea salt together in a bowl.

2. Heat the infused coconut oil in the microwave on medium power until just melted.

3. Cool the melted oil slightly (until 140°F or cooler) and stir in the peppermint, sweet orange, and rosemary essential oils.

4. Pour the oil into the salts and stir well until the oil is evenly distributed. Mix in the dried rose petals, if using.

5. Transfer to an airtight container.

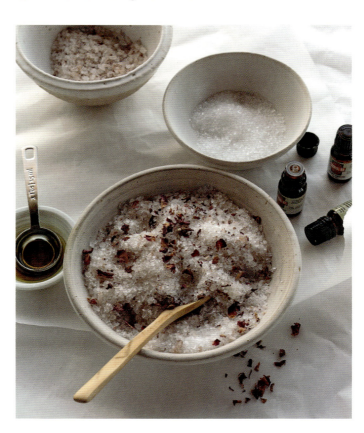

Suppositories for
Vaginal and Anal Application

People use cannabis suppositories for everything from period cramps to vaginal dryness, or anal suppositories for inflamed bowels and other ailments residing in that area. Some use them to enhance sex, though a less messy option may be cannabis intimacy oil (see the next section, "Personal Lubricants and Sensual Oils"). Suppositories containing THC can even be good for combating hip or lower back pain, ulcerative colitis, or endometriosis-related pain. But beware: Unlike with other cannabis-infused topicals, you *can* get high by using a vaginal suppository that contains THC. However, according to Jamie Evans, it's a different kind of high. "You're not going to get the same head high," she reports. Part of the reason for this is that cannabinoids that enter your body vaginally or rectally are not metabolized via the liver. Gretchen Miller, founder and CEO of California-based luxury cannabis brand Kiskanu, says that for this reason, you can usually take higher doses of THC via a suppository than you could orally. "I have had numerous clients who can't take THC edibles at doses higher than 2 milligrams but could handle my 50-milligram THC suppository and found great relief from it, feeling relaxed and able to still perform at work," she says.

There's some contradictory research regarding the absorption rate of cannabinoids in this family of products, especially anal suppositories. Some studies indicate that suppositories yield the highest rate of absorption, while others found it to be among the lowest, even indicating that THC cannot be absorbed through rectal walls unless bonded to a separate molecule. An explanation for this could be in the way the cannabinoids are delivered. Evidently, oils are not well absorbed through the rectum. Several studies now indicate the ability to absorb THC through the suppository method can be achieved by first processing THC into THC-HS, a water-soluble form, which is promising for folks who are looking for the benefits of THC without inhaling it or eating it. And even if the THC doesn't absorb through the walls of the rectum, there's plenty of anecdotal support for its use to treat gastrointestinal and gynecological disorders.

Kiskanu makes a calendula and coconut oil–based suppository with 50 milligrams of THC and 15 milligrams of CBD in each one, as well as a CBD version that you can buy online or at Anthropologie and Saks Fifth Avenue. Foria, also based in California, makes both a CBD version and a THC + CBD version. It's best if you store the suppositories in the fridge so they won't melt as soon as you insert them. Both companies also advise that you lie down for at least twenty minutes after insertion, to allow the medicine to seep in before gravity does its thing.

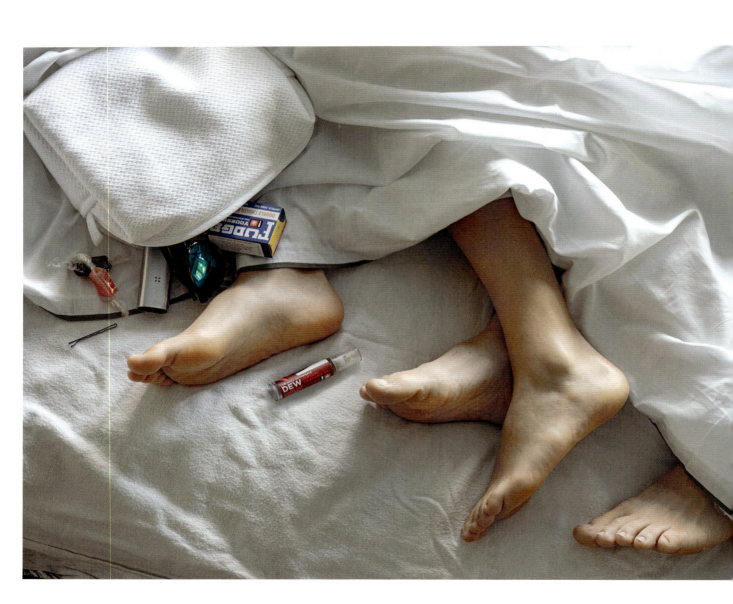

Personal Lubricants and Sensual Oils

Cannabis lubricants, sensual oils, or sprays will keep your sensitive areas lubricated with the added bonus of increased sensitivity and more intense and frequent orgasms. Yes please!

These products promote arousal during sex and amplify orgasms. Oh my. Foria's Awaken, which contains broad-spectrum CBD and nine plant-based aphrodisiacs, including cacao, cardamom, and kava kava, gets high marks for sparking pleasure while reducing dryness and discomfort—and smelling like chocolate mint. Foria also makes Pleasure, a "natural arousal lube" with THC, but it's sold only in California and Colorado dispensaries. The product won a *Cosmopolitan* Sexcellence award in 2019 and receives rave reviews on its website. One woman wrote, "Y'all need to make this stuff in bulk, load it in an airplane, and start spraying it over the entire world population because this stuff could bring world peace. HOLY WOW. Best sex ever after just one use."

Empower BodyCare makes a sought-after sensual oil spray called 4Play. "You know how when you're fooling around with someone and you get so turned on?" says Celia Behar, who runs the popular mommy blog Lil' Mamas. "It does that for you. It makes it so that you get crazy turned on. And then it just enhances everything. Sex. Everything." Behar has gone so far as to promote the product on her blog, giving moms a discount code. One Oregon woman wrote to her and said, "It's like my vagina got the munchies for my husband's [BLEEP]." And she didn't say "ears."

As with any product containing THC, it's important to play around with dosage. If you use it once and don't feel anything, try a few more sprays (or applications) next time. Behar had a friend who was going through menopause and used 4Play, and she said it didn't work. "The next time, she ended up needing to use five or six sprays, and she realized that it depended on her metabolism. One night she wrote me and said, 'I overdosed myself with 4Play.' She was like, 'I feel like a cat in heat. I'm walking up to furniture and rubbing myself on it.'" You've been warned!

White Sage and
Rosemary Massage Oil

Yield: 8 ounces

This massage oil is heavenly. THC and CBD add anti-inflammatory and pain-relieving properties to the blend, resulting in a massage oil that will leave you feeling balanced and relaxed.

2 ounces infused coconut oil

6 ounces sweet almond oil, olive oil, avocado oil, or hemp oil

20 drops rosemary essential oil

20 drops white sage essential oil

Rosemary sprigs for garnish, optional

White sage sprigs for garnish, optional

1. Place the infused coconut oil in a heatproof glass jar. Fill a saucepan with a couple of inches of water and bring to a simmer over medium-high heat. Place the jar in the pan. Heat until melted.

2. While the coconut oil is melting, set up the container for the massage oil. Fill the container with the sweet almond oil, the rosemary and white sage essential oils, and the rosemary and white sage sprigs, if using.

3. Once the coconut oil has melted, remove the jar from the pan and pour the coconut oil into the container with the other oils. Stir, shake, or swirl the container well to combine.

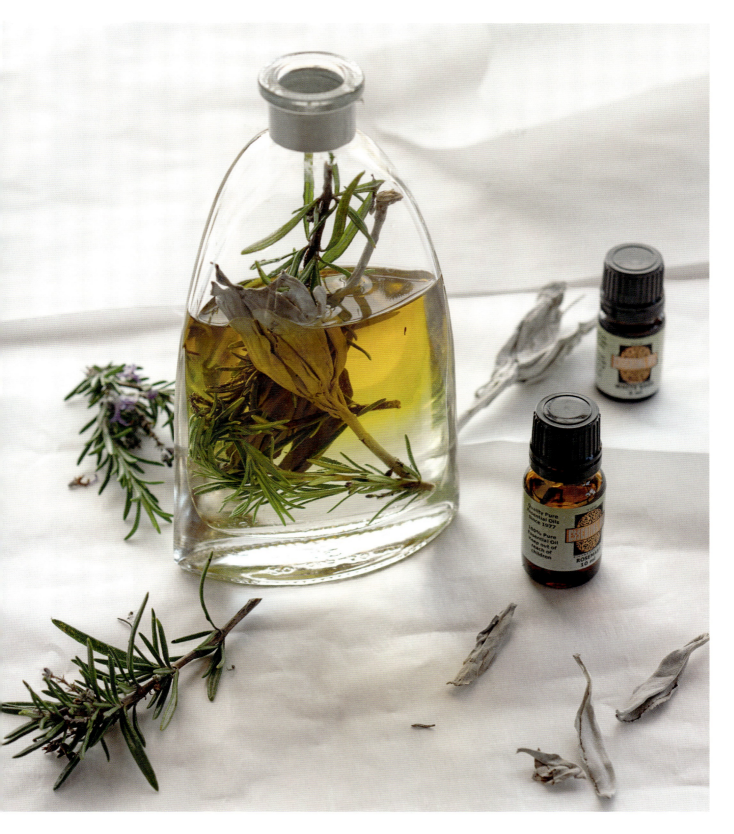

Lemon and Mint Lip Balm

Yield: 2 ½ ounces

This topical crosses over into the edible category, and that is just fine with me. If you're like me, you might find yourself reapplying every 15 minutes, resulting in lush lips and elevated spirits. How many other lip balms can you say that about?

1 tablespoon beeswax pellets

3 tablespoons sweet almond oil, olive oil, avocado oil, or hemp oil

1 tablespoon canna-coconut oil (see Canna Oil)

10 drops lemon essential oil

5 drops peppermint essential oil

1. Place the beeswax, sweet almond oil, and infused coconut oil in a heatproof glass jar. Fill a saucepan with a couple of inches of water and bring it to a simmer over medium-high heat. Place the jar in the pan. Stir periodically until all ingredients have melted. Turn the heat down if the water begins to boil.

2. Once everything has melted, remove the jar from the pan and allow it to cool slightly, until the contents of the jar are less than 140°F/60°C. Add the lemon and peppermint essential oils and stir well to combine.

3. While the mixture is still liquid, pour it into your desired containers. We used ten ¼-ounce glass lip balm containers.

A Note on DIY Topical Recipes

With a batch of infused coconut oil, you can make a wide range of wellness items. We put together a few recipes in these pages to help get you started. As with any topical, a patch test should be performed before use, especially if you have sensitive skin. These recipes can be made with oil infused with THC or CBD-rich flower. Feel free to swap any of the essential oils for a customized experience.

Pink Peppercorn and Orange Salve

Yield: 9 ounces

Salves are a simple, soothing topical that can be easily tailored to your desired use. I like to use pink peppercorn essential oil for its stimulating and pain-relieving properties, and I use sweet orange essential oil for its uplifting and anti-inflammatory qualities.

2 tablespoons beeswax pellets

½ cup infused coconut oil

½ cup sweet almond oil, olive oil, avocado oil, or hemp oil

10 drops pink peppercorn essential oil

5 drops sweet orange essential oil

Pink peppercorns for garnish, optional

Orange peel for garnish, optional

1. Place the beeswax, coconut oil, and sweet almond oil in a heatproof glass jar. Fill a saucepan with a couple of inches of water and bring to a simmer over medium-high heat. Place the jar in the pan. Stir periodically until all ingredients have melted. Turn the heat down if the water begins to boil.

2. Once everything has melted, remove the jar from the pan and allow it to cool slightly, until the contents of the jar are less than 140°F/ 60°C. Add the peppercorn and sweet orange essential oils and stir well to combine.

3. While the mixture is still liquid, pour it into your desired container(s); we used five 2-ounce wide-mouth metal containers. Stir in the peppercorn and orange peel garnish, if using.

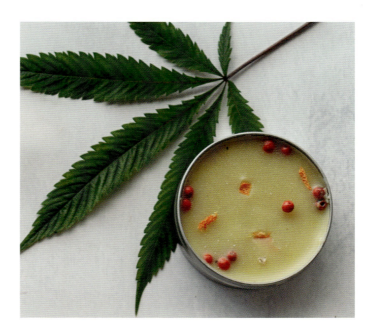

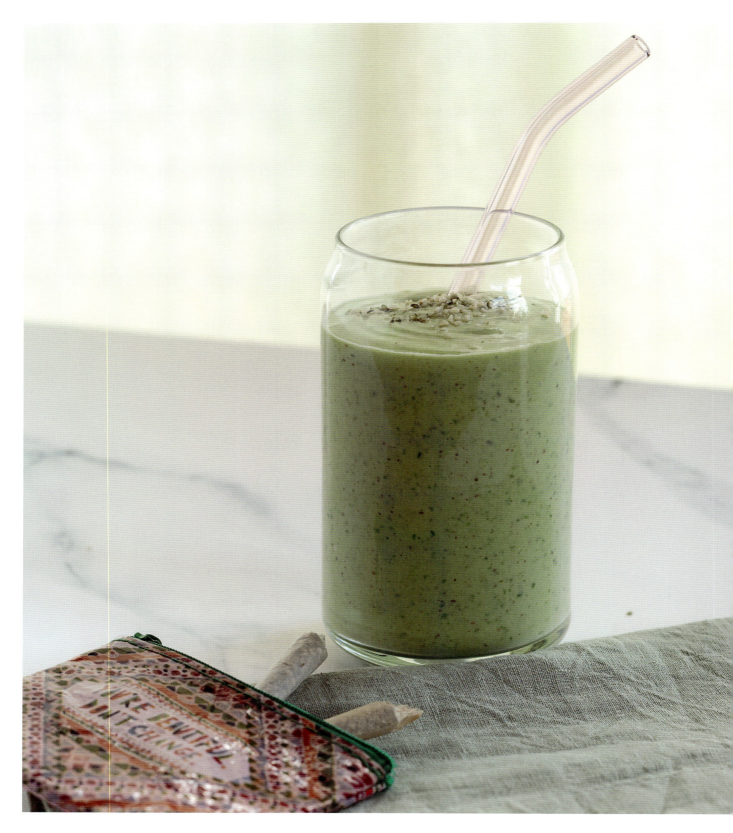

Green Smoothie

Yield: 2¹/₂ cups | Serving: 1¹/₄ cup
THC: 5 milligrams per serving (10 milligrams total)

I never thought I would enjoy drinking avocado anything. I also didn't know how healthy the avocado is. This drink is fire! Get a ripe avocado (yields to gentle pressure) and give it a whirl in the blender with the rest of the ingredients. Sometimes I wonder if a savory version of this smoothie that includes all the stuff that goes in guacamole would be good. Why not experiment a little and see what you think?

1 ripe avocado

1¹/₂ cups almond milk

¹/₂ cup almond butter

1–2 tablespoons honey, to taste

2 teaspoons hemp or chia seeds

1. Combine the avocado, almond milk, almond butter, and honey in a blender. Process until smooth.

2. Divide between two glasses and top each with 1 teaspoon of either hemp or chia seeds.

So Pretty Pink Smoothie Shots

Yield: 32 ounces | Serving: 4 ounces

CBD: 7.5 milligrams per serving (60 milligrams total)

For the last few months I have been walking with a small group of fairly lazy people. I'm not much of an exercise fan, so getting outside with a group of people works best for me. I guess it's a misery loves company thing. These are the CBD smoothie shots our walking group takes. It's a low dose, but it does the trick.

2 cups almond milk or any kind of milk

1 cup strawberries, trimmed and rinsed

½ banana, sliced and frozen

1 cup pineapple chunks

1–2 tablespoons honey or agave, to taste

2 tablespoons hemp-infused coconut oil

2 tablespoons hemp seeds

1 cup freeze-dried strawberries, chopped

1. Combine all of the ingredients in a blender. Process until smooth. Divide among 8 glasses and garnish with chopped, freeze-dried strawberries. Drink immediately.

2. Store any leftovers in the refrigerator, making sure you put your smoothie through the blender again before re-serving.

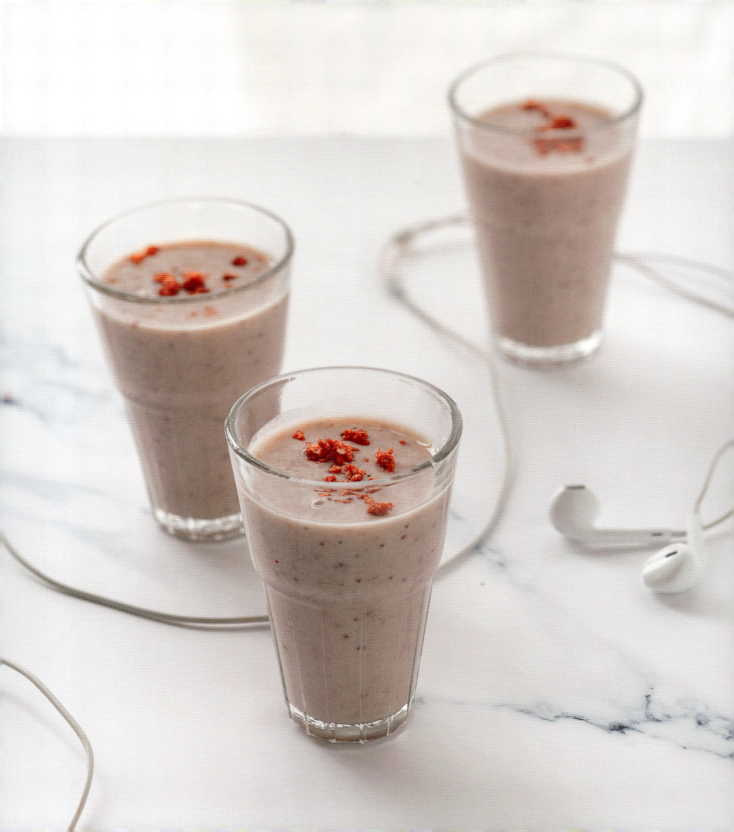

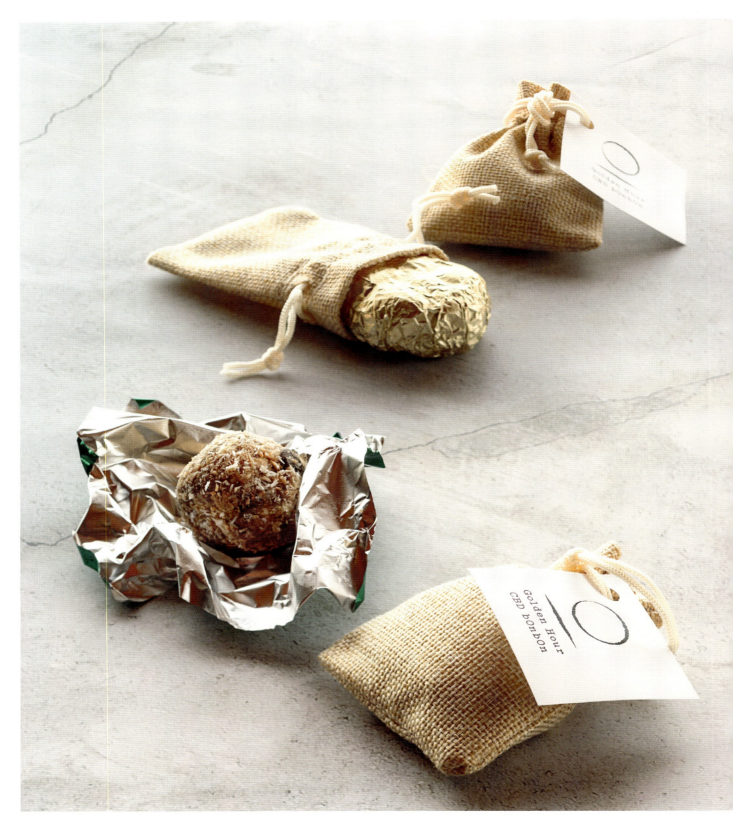

Easy Edible Energy Balls

Yield: 20 balls | Serving: 1 ball

THC: 5 milligrams per serving (100 milligrams total)

There is a beautiful wellness studio in Portland named Golden Hour. It's all about health, beauty, and balance. On the CBD side of our company, Laurie + MaryJane, we create these energy balls for a hit of goodness and a healthy indulgence.

1 cup old-fashioned rolled oats

½ cup almond butter

½ cup hemp seeds

½ cup dark chocolate chips

10 teaspoons infused coconut oil

¼ cup honey

1 tablespoon chia seeds

2 teaspoons vanilla extract

½ cup shredded unsweetened coconut, toasted

1. Combine the oats, almond butter, hemp seeds, chocolate chips, infused coconut oil, honey, chia seeds, and vanilla in the bowl of a food processor. Process until the oats are finely ground and everything is well blended. Place the mixture in the fridge for 1 hour.

2. Remove the mixture from the fridge and roll into twenty 1-inch balls. Place the toasted coconut on a plate and roll the balls into the coconut, pressing as you roll to adhere the coconut. If you have leftovers, store them in an airtight container in the refrigerator.

CBD Granola

Yield: 6 cups | Serving: ¹/₂ cup

CBD: 5 milligrams per serving (60 milligrams total)

———

You can buy Laurie + MaryJane CBD granola online, or simply follow this similar recipe. Obviously, I can't share our company's exact recipe, but this one is pretty darn great. Remember that any recipe can be made with either CBD or THC, or a combination of both. People love the combination as it offers the best of both cannabis worlds.

4 cups old-fashioned rolled oats

1 cup almonds, roughly chopped

¹/₃ cup toasted walnuts, coarsely chopped

¹/₃ cup chopped dried apricots

¹/₄ cup dried cranberries

¹/₂ cup chia seeds

2 teaspoons ground cinnamon

¹/₈ teaspoon ground nutmeg

Pinch salt

²/₃ cup maple syrup

2 tablespoons infused coconut oil

2 teaspoons vanilla

1. Heat the oven to 300°F/149°C.

2. Line a lipped baking sheet with parchment paper. In a bowl, combine the oats, almonds, walnuts, apricots, cranberries, chia seeds, cinnamon, nutmeg, and salt.

3. In a separate bowl, combine the maple syrup, infused oil, and vanilla. Pour over the oat mixture and mix well. Spread the mixture evenly on the baking sheet.

4. Bake, stirring occasionally, for 35–40 minutes until light to medium golden brown. Cool completely before breaking up the large clusters and storing in an airtight container.

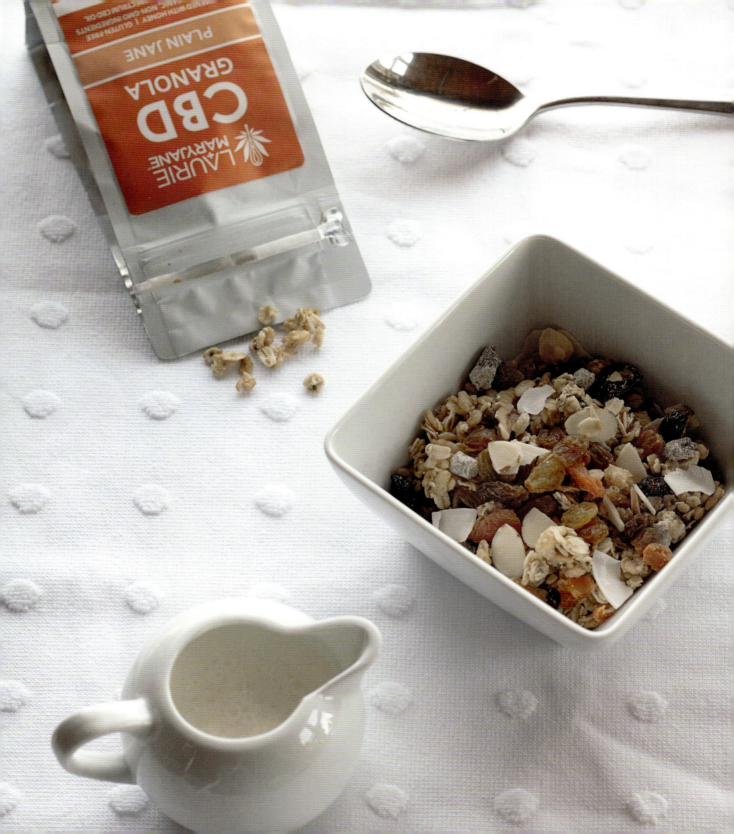

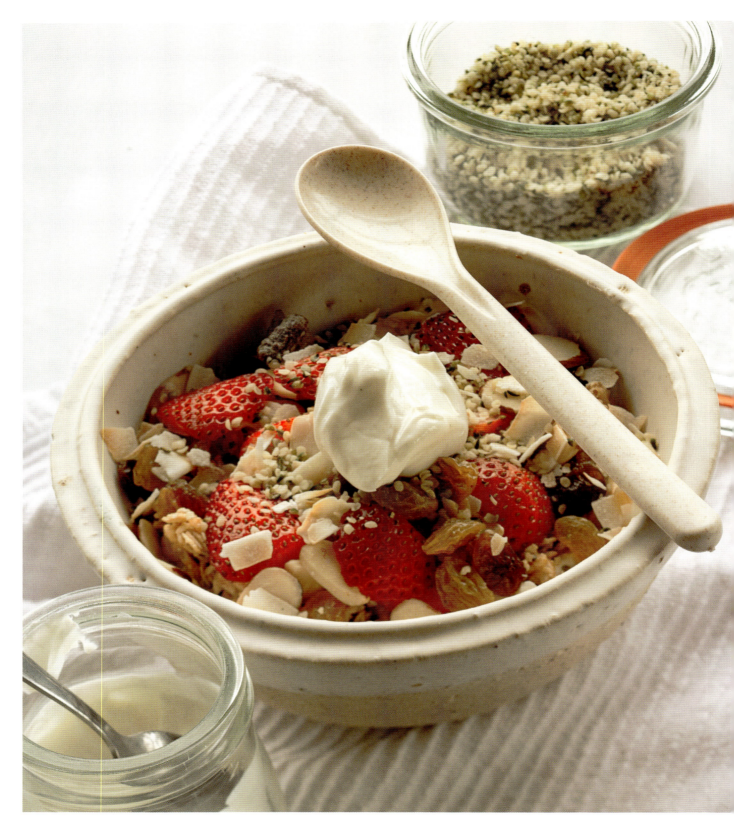

Granola Bowl

Yield: 1 bowl | Serving: 1 bowl | CBD: 5 milligrams

What a terrific way to start the day! Use a serving of granola from the previous page, and this bowl comes together in moments. Feel free to change the fruit or the nuts to help make this recipe your own. I've made this dish with ricotta and cottage cheese as well, and it's equally delicious. Cottage cheese is underestimated in this world.

$2/3$ cup vanilla yogurt

$1/2$ cup granola

2 tablespoons yellow raisins

3 strawberries, trimmed and sliced

2 tablespoons toasted coconut flakes

2 tablespoons sliced almonds

1 tablespoon hemp seeds

1. This is all about the layering. Start with the yogurt and layer the ingredients as you desire. There is no wrong way to go here. No matter how you layer your ingredients, you're destined to end up with a wonderful bowl of morning (or any time) deliciousness.

Golden Milk

Yield: 2 cups | Serving: 1 cup

THC: 5 milligrams per serving (10 milligrams total)

This soothing beverage is often one of my nighttime pleasures. Turmeric aids with digestion and has impressive anti-inflammatory properties. Ginger and cinnamon also contribute to this creamy and warm nutritional powerhouse. This infusion will help you get through the night.

1 cup canned coconut milk

1 cup almond milk

1–2 tablespoons maple syrup, to taste

2 teaspoons turmeric

½ teaspoon ground ginger, plus more for garnish

¼ teaspoon ground cinnamon, plus more for garnish

1 teaspoon infused coconut oil

1. In a medium saucepan, combine the coconut milk, almond milk, maple syrup, turmeric, ginger, and cinnamon and heat on low. The mixture should be hot but should not come to a boil.

2. Whisk in the infused oil and divide between two cups. If desired, sprinkle with additional ginger and/or cinnamon.

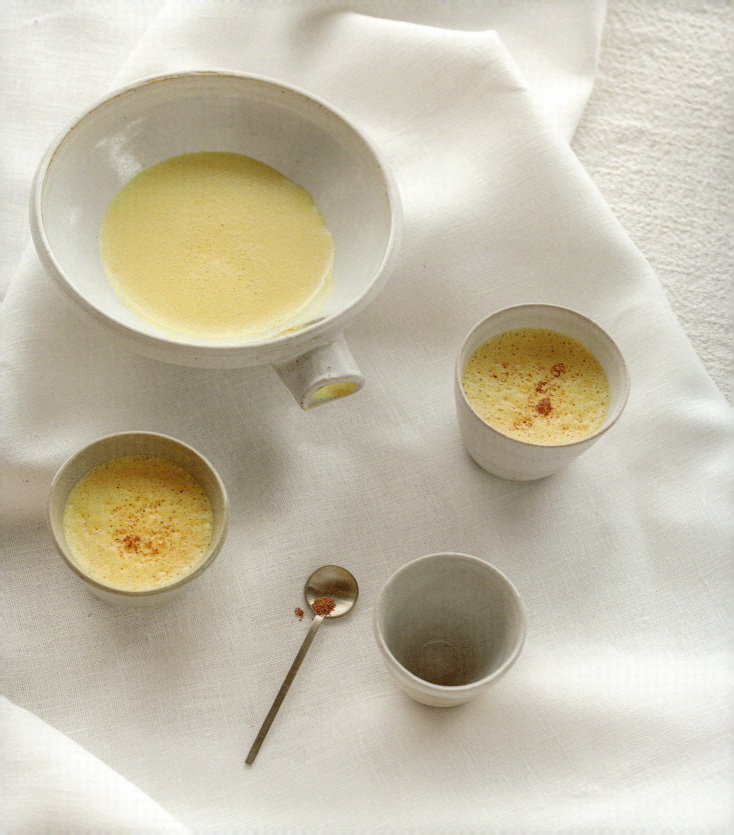

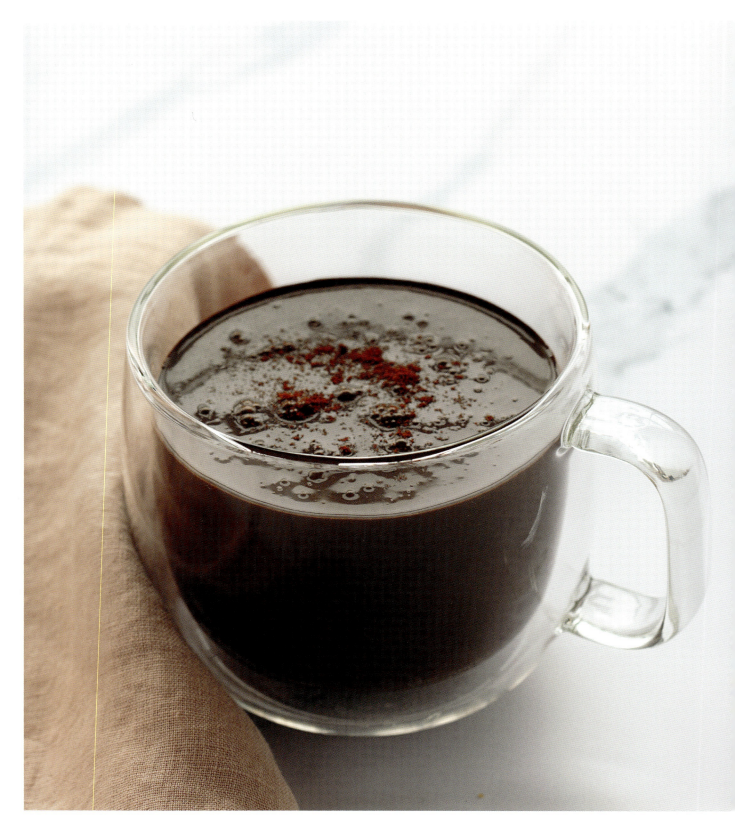

Way Hot Chocolate

Yield: 2 large mugs | Serving: 1 large mug

THC: 5 milligrams per serving (10 milligrams total)

This is a special-occasion hot chocolate. It's decadent. The half-and-half adds a velvety quality to this libation, and the brown sugar brings a hint of caramel. You won't taste the cannabis, but relax—you'll feel it soon enough. If you want to get extra crazy, spray a piece of parchment paper with non-stick cooking spray, and then cover it with mini marshmallows, placing them in groups of 5 to 8. Microwave for 10 to 20 seconds. The marshmallows will melt and get a little caramelized, and they'll taste delicious in your hot chocolate.

1¼ cups milk

1 cup half-and-half

1 tablespoon brown sugar

4 ounces dark chocolate, chopped

2 teaspoons vanilla

2 teaspoons canna-butter

1 teaspoon instant coffee powder

Pinch salt

1. In a medium saucepan, heat the milk, half-and-half, and brown sugar to very hot but not boiling. Remove from the heat. Add the chocolate. Stir to melt.

2. When the chocolate is fully melted, add the vanilla, canna-butter, coffee powder, and salt.

3. Whisk well.

Thai Tea

Yield: 2 cups | Serving: 1 cup

THC: 5 milligrams per serving (10 milligrams total)

Although I adore the color of Thai tea, I was bummed to learn that the color is derived from food coloring. I have removed the food coloring and added a dose of turmeric, a nutritional powerhouse spice that is a strong antioxidant and has significant anti-inflammatory properties. And it's pretty and natural. What a lovely drink it is.

2 cups water

2 tablespoons loose black tea or 3 tea bags

¼ cup sugar

1 star anise

1 smashed cardamom pod

7 ounces condensed milk

1 teaspoon canna-butter

2 teaspoons vanilla

1 teaspoon turmeric

Mint leaves or lime wedges, for garnish, optional

1. Bring 2 cups of water to a boil in a small saucepan. Remove from the heat and add the tea. Allow the tea to steep for 3 minutes, then strain.

2. Add the sugar, star anise, cardamom, condensed milk, canna-butter, vanilla, and turmeric to the strained tea. Allow it to come to room temperature. Fill 2 glasses with ice and strain the mixture into the glasses. Garnish with mint leaves or lime wedges.

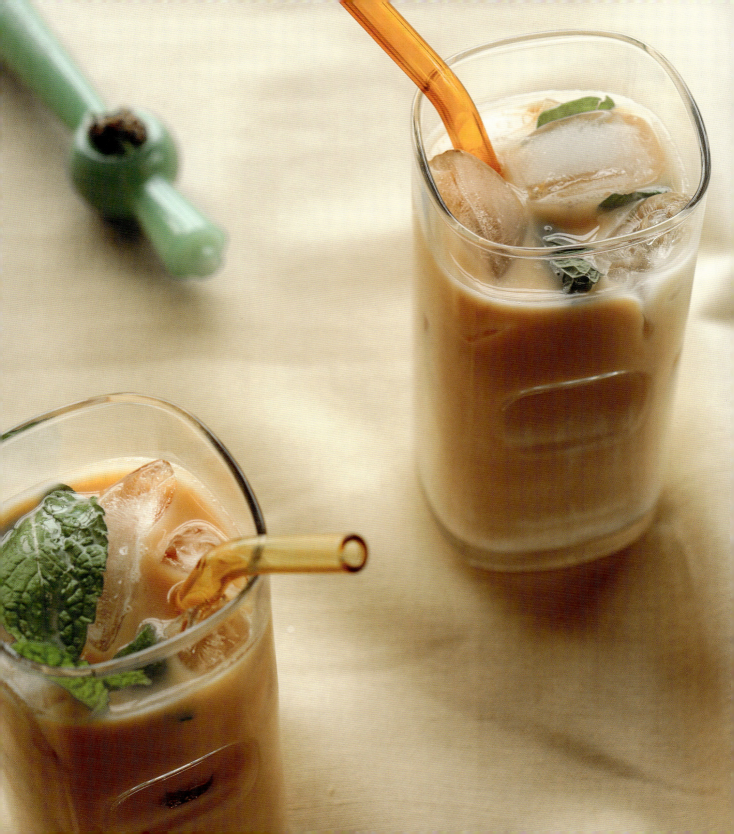

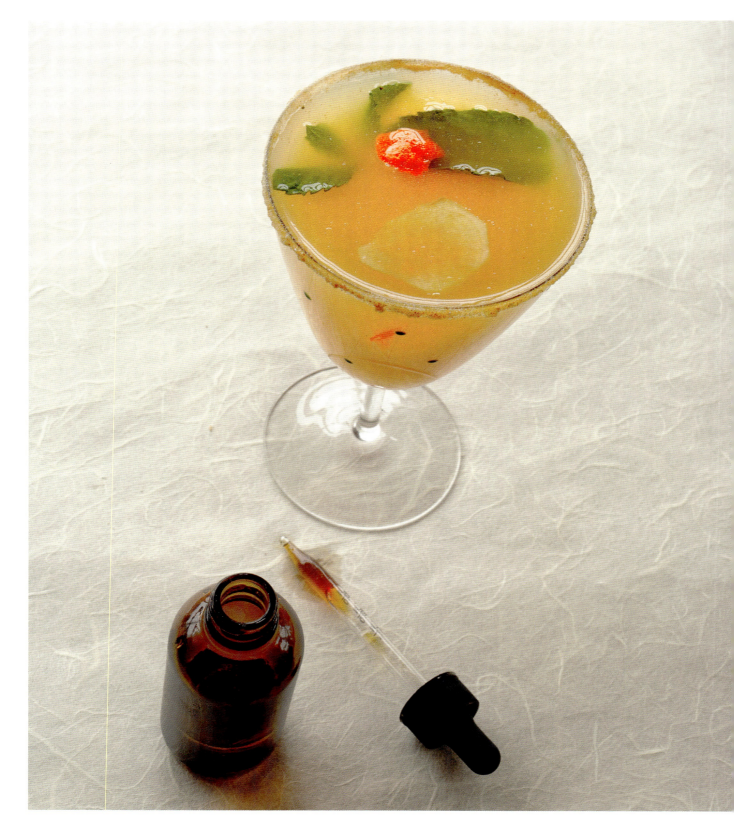

Pineapple Ginger CBD Cocktail

Yield: 4 glasses | Serving: 1 glass

THC: 5 milligrams per serving (20 milligrams total)

Adding CBD to an alcoholic drink is a double delight. I'm not a fan of mixing THC and alcohol, but this non-psychoactive combination is a winner. It's also gorgeous, not that looks matter.

¼ cup lime juice

3 tablespoons sugar

2 teaspoons ground ginger

2 cups pineapple juice

4 thin slices fresh peeled ginger

4 thin orange slices or segments

12 mint leaves

2 teaspoons CBD tincture

4 teaspoons grenadine

1 cup sparkling wine (I use Prosecco)

1. Place 4 glasses on your work surface. Place the lime juice on a small plate or saucer.

2. In a small bowl, combine the sugar and the ginger. Run the rim of each glass through the lime juice and then the sugar mixture, forming a sugared rim on each glass.

3. Divide the pineapple juice among the glasses. Add a piece of ginger, a slice of orange, and 3 mint leaves to each of the glasses. Divide the tincture and the grenadine among the glasses.

4. Just before serving, divide the Prosecco among the glasses. Cheers!

Q & A
WITH OLIVIA ALEXANDER,
FOUNDER AND CEO OF CALIFORNIA'S KUSH QUEEN

By the time she launched luxury cannabis brand Kush Queen in 2015, Olivia Alexander had already founded a cannabis marketing company and a crystal vape pen business—and she had amassed a loyal social media following. Her first official Kush Queen products were a line of cannabis bath bombs, which became an overnight hit. In the five years since, she's expanded her product line to include lotions, lubes, gummies, and tinctures. Alexander, thirty-one, feels lucky to be in the cannabis industry, spreading the word about this powerful plant. "This is going to be the future. CBD and cannabinoids are going to inhabit everything that exists—from fashion to experiences," she says. Alexander, who was diagnosed with bipolar disorder when she was eighteen, says cannabis has helped her with mental health, sleep, and more. As such, she sees it as her mission to integrate cannabis into the lives of others—one bath bomb at a time.

Why bath bombs?

My philosophy of changing people's minds about cannabis is that you find something really friendly or familiar. People don't like change, especially the types of people who I'm trying to convert to cannabis (they are type A personalities, not stoners). You can't convince those people to smoke it in a pipe or roll it in a joint. That is so scary to people. The bath bomb is so approachable. And also, it's extremely effective. When you submerge yourself in a body of water, there are already health benefits. The skin is the biggest organ. The bath bomb is really very smart. It's the perfect way to take on cannabinoids. Once they're into the bath bombs, that's when we hit them with all the other products!

🌿 Can you get high from bath bombs?

No. The particle size is too big to enter the bloodstream. People say they've gotten high from it, but that's a placebo effect. I think that's another reason we became so big in California—because some people are terrified of getting high. They're terrified! They don't want to change their consciousness. Whereas Millennials and Gen Xers, they're like, "Where can I go to change my consciousness?"

🌿 What other Kush Queen products are hugely popular?

The two other products that are our bread and butter are Ignite CBD lubricant—which is a real lube and it absorbs right in due to nanoparticles—and the Melt pain lotion, which is a combination of essential oils and nanoparticles. It activates the area, and the CBD goes right into the bloodstream and targets the pain. People go insane for the Melt.

🌿 You do a lot of collaborations with other companies. Tell me more!

Bellacures, which has seven salons in the Los Angeles area, started doing manicures and pedicures with our products. Again: It's familiar. If you're a woman, you have gotten a lot of manis and pedis. When you get one while you're soaking your feet in CBD—you're really absorbing it. Then they massage your legs with our Renew sugar scrub, and then Melt away pain relief lotion. With [New York-based fashion house] Alice + Olivia, we're doing a 200-milligram bath bomb with vetiver, sandalwood, and lavender. It's a crazy sleep combination! And a bubble bath with a hint of lavender and then a basic body lotion. Creative director and CEO Stacey Bendet is such a She-ro. She's a fashionista, and she loves our gummies and tinctures.

🌿 What's next?

I just launched my CBD makeup line. It's called KINGDM Cosmetics. We're starting with a primer, Foto Blur, and then a setting spray and foundations.

⚜ It seems like you do a lot of CBD products!

Yeah, now we're predominantly a CBD company, which breaks my heart. The truth is that legal cannabis is not a legit industry in California, because the black market is so powerful here. It takes so much enforcement to really shut down the black market. When you tax a person 40 percent [to buy legal cannabis products], you'll never be able to shut down the black market.

⚜ How did you get into the cannabis space?

I got my start in 2007 with the Crystal Cult—crystal vaporizer pens and rhinestone accessories. Back then, I spent all my money on weed. I bought products. I remember walking into a dispensary and seeing the finished chocolate bars and my heart shook.

⚜ How does Kush Queen help people incorporate cannabis into their lifestyle?

All I'm trying to do is convince people that it's not just CBD, but all cannabinoids, that are good. Sure, we're making money, but we're opening up access to women who are still not using CBD. People need this stuff, they really do. At the end of the day, it's so powerful.

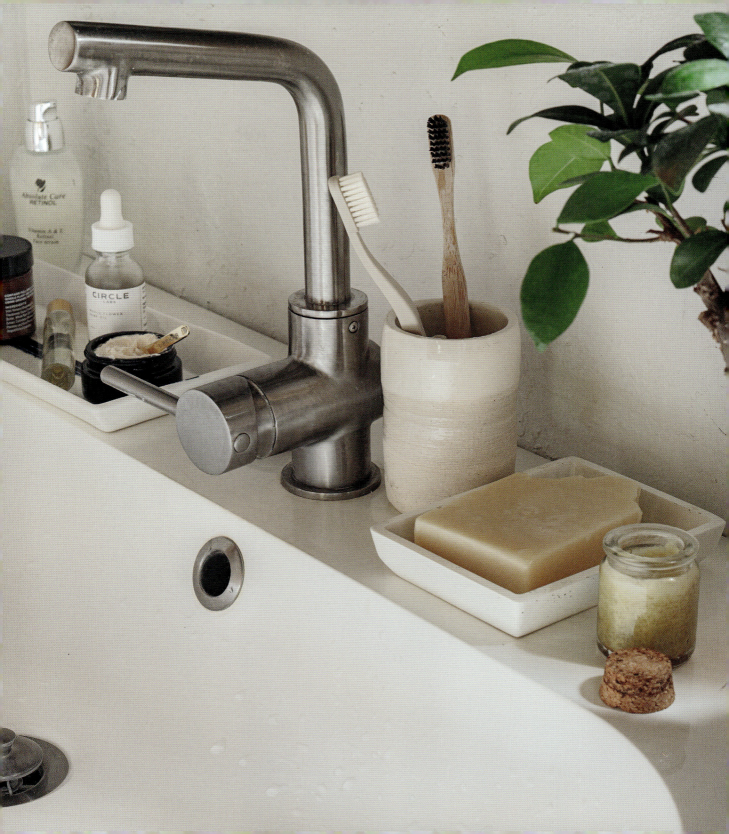

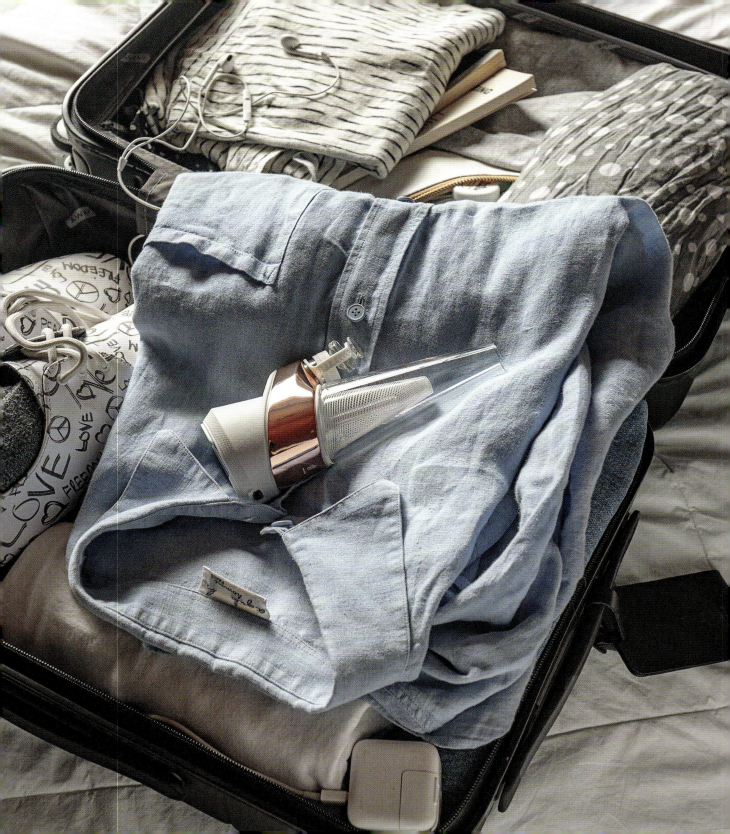

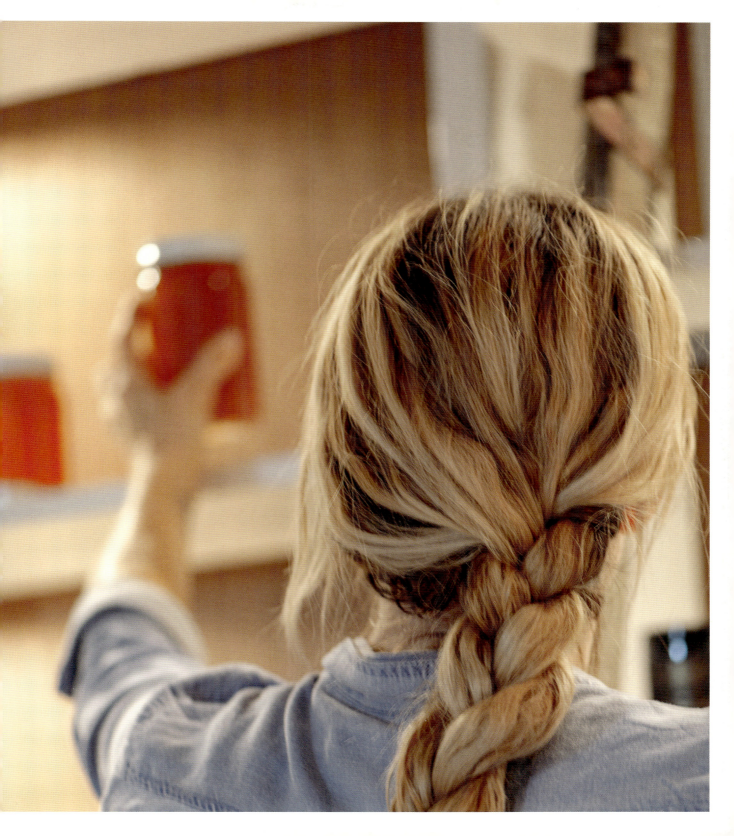

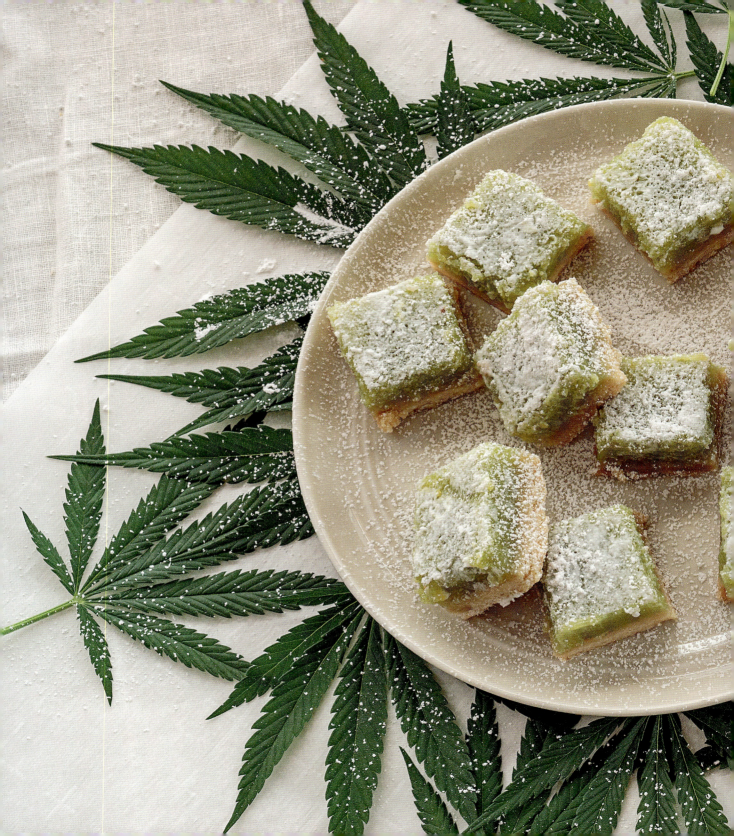

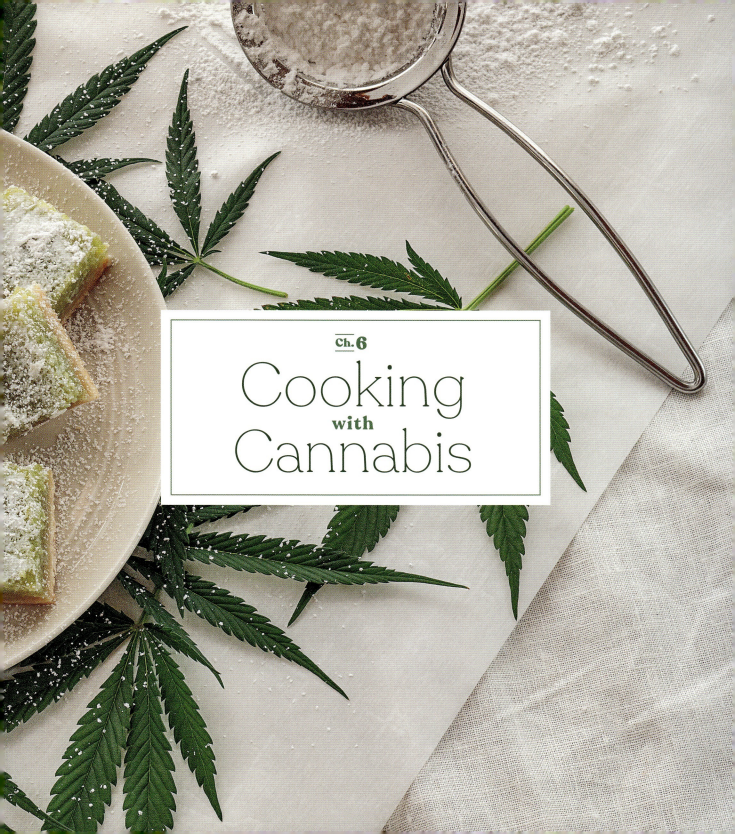

Ch. 6

Cooking
with
Cannabis

A couple of weeks ago I attended a cannabis dinner party celebrating the birthday of a friend who has a large cannabis farm in southern Oregon. Not being much of a cook, the birthday boy/chef for the day grilled me ahead of time on the how-tos. We planned the menu together: three courses with 10 milligrams of THC and 20 milligrams of CBD, per person, total. Things were looking promising. The cannabis flower's potency was tested at a lab so I was able to give explicit instructions to my buddy regarding dosing, arguably the most important piece in the puzzle of a successful cannabis-infused dining experience. None of the recipes were too challenging, and my plan was to get there in the early afternoon to help out.

Entering the kitchen, I was comforted by the familiar aroma of an infused tomato sauce gently simmering on the stove; dotting the countertop were bowls of ingredients, along with a bunch of handwritten notes he had taken during our meal-planning Skype sessions. My friend's foray into the world of cannabis cooking looked and smelled promising.

Not so fast.

Unfortunately, my buddy had made a classic mistake and was suffering the consequences. He had been cooking since morning, and he had overtasted. Although we had planned a low-dose meal, the frequent tastes of this and that had led him to ingest way more cannabis than he could tolerate. I found him lying on his bed, bleary-eyed and laughing rather hysterically. He was wasted. He didn't feel bad, but he was too far gone to be able to follow the recipes. Lying in bed for the next five hours was all he could manage—a forced vacation of sorts. Eventually, once he felt okay sitting upright, he completely emptied his dresser and color coordinated his wardrobe. While all this was going on, I cooked the rest of the meal, and by 7:00 p.m., we were both ready to party.

During recipe testing, continuous tasting can add up. I've been there. Not unlike wine, lots of little tastes can result in unintentionally overdoing it. I am not at all sure that I warned him about this outcome. Bad, bad Laurie! That is a mistake I've vowed to never repeat. So consider this your warning: Taste testing adds up, so don't overdo it.

There are a couple of other rules that need to be followed if you want to have a successful cannabis-infused dining experience. The most important rule when entertaining is to never overdose your guests. In addition to being the most important rule, it is also the most difficult to follow. While the cannabis experience can differ drastically from one person to another, it is only pleasant when you have not consumed too much.

Entertaining

Over the years, we have had many cannabis dinner parties, some amazing, some not so great, some even written about in *Vogue* and *The New Yorker*, if you can believe it. We are still finding ways to enhance the experience and keep everyone in a pleasant state. Mary and I have developed some house rules to make sure everyone has a good time. Not crazy or unreasonable rules, just sensible rules that make for a much better experience, especially for me. Our first few events were fine and fun, but there was one problem that I kept running into, and it made the dinners a 7 instead of a 10. The problem was that I got stoned. I said I wouldn't, I said that to myself, and to others, but when the vaporizer came out, I got in line. I love a party, and I love cannabis. But a good host needs to keep their wits about them, and that did not always happen in my case.

I have since changed my cannabis dinner party etiquette. No edibles and no smoking or vaping until dessert is served. Then I will succumb to my pleasures and indulge in a thing or two. I have to confess that I seem to be kind of obnoxious when I get high. Not mean or aggressive—I just don't shut up, and I talk about how high I am. Then I say I will stop, but I don't. Since I know how I am when I'm high, I've adjusted my behavior accordingly. Here are some basic rules that I follow to make sure everyone has a good time:

🌿 Find out about guests' allergies and cannabis experience. I live in Portland, Oregon, where every third person in the city has to have a food allergy.

🌿 Plan a menu that has a THC limit of 8 to 10 milligrams. The whole meal equals 10 milligrams THC, or lower.

🌿 Label everything. Label everything. Label everything!

🌿 Offer infused sauces, dips, or garnishes (like croutons) for those who have a higher tolerance. And always have non-infused food for people who don't want to indulge. You can ignore them, but you have to feed them.

🌿 Encourage people not to go overboard. Less is more.

🌿 Don't let friends drive home under the influence. Make a plan.

🌿 Spend at least twenty minutes sitting together and listening to music. No screens, and no phones or TV—they can all be a bit too hypnotic when you're under the influence. We've always found that a good album can enliven the group and put you in the right frame of mind.

🌿 This should go without being said, but I'm going to say it here anyway: Never give cannabis to children (anyone under eighteen), or pregnant women.

🌿 Eat yummy food. In moderation.

In my kitchen there are jars with infused items that I can toss in a recipe to infuse at the last minute:

- Croutons
- Chocolate sauce
- Caramel sauce
- Spice blends
- "Herb" and herb-infused olive oil
- Frozen cubes of infused pesto
- Compound butter
- Infused nut mix
- Infused nut butters

Experimenting to Find Your Ideal Dosage

A single serving size for any given recipe in this book is 1 teaspoon of canna-butter or canna-oil, which contains a dose of 5 milligrams of THC. In our tests, this dose was enough for most occasional cannabis users to feel minor psychoactivity. As you begin to experiment with THC-infused cooking, we suggest giving yourself five days to experiment, increasing your THC dose by 2 to 3 milligrams each day. For users who are relatively new to cannabis, we suggest starting with a dose as low as 2 milligrams of THC, or lower if you're a total newbie. Keep in mind, it is always better to experience no effect than to overdo it.

When I speak in front of groups, people always have stories to share about that time, in college, when they ate an infused brownie and were messed up for hours. That's not a dangerous place to be, but it can be pretty miserable. As you experiment with cannabis and edibles, here are a few important tips to follow that will keep you from running into trouble:

🌿 Cannabis consumed orally can affect the body more powerfully than cannabis consumed by inhalation. We recommend starting with a 2-milligram serving size or even less for your first few times, until you better understand how the THC level affects you.

🌿 It can take anywhere from forty-five minutes to two hours (or even longer) to feel the effects of cannabis consumed in edible form. It is impossible to know how edibles will affect you personally until you experience them, so be cautious and responsible when getting started.

🌿 Until you know how cannabis affects you, you should try edibles on a full stomach, or eat something without cannabis in it at the same time that you eat your edible.

🌱 Edibles with a higher fat content will generally have a longer-lasting effect compared to edibles with a high sugar content, which will pass through your system more quickly.

For those of you who have the benefit of obtaining cannabis with potency results (you know the percentages of THC and CBD), you'll be able to calibrate your infusions with confidence. (Quick reminder: The potency of a cannabis strain is presented as a percentage of the weight of THC to the weight of the plant material. So a 1-gram bud that is 20 percent THC will contain 200 milligrams of THC.)

When I speak to groups of current or curious edible enthusiasts, I suggest starting with a dose as low as 2 milligrams of THC. Although, for some people, 2 milligrams of THC can even be too much. (I'm looking at you, Dan Pashman.) People who regularly take CBD may be able to start a bit higher; 5 to 7 milligrams is a good place to begin.

With a little patience, you can incrementally increase your daily dose slowly until you zero in on the potency that is right for you. For example, give yourself five days and increase your dose by 2 to 3 milligrams of THC each day. For most folks, following these steps will help you find your edible potency number, which tells you how many milligrams it takes to get you feeling good but not wasted. And yes, over time your potency might change. If that happens, just incrementally adjust your dose using the same steps we've just laid out.

This is a plan that is worth following. It takes a bit of patience, but please work with us here. The high you get from eating edibles is different than what you may have experienced from smoking cannabis. It comes on slowly, involves both body and mind, and can last for several hours.

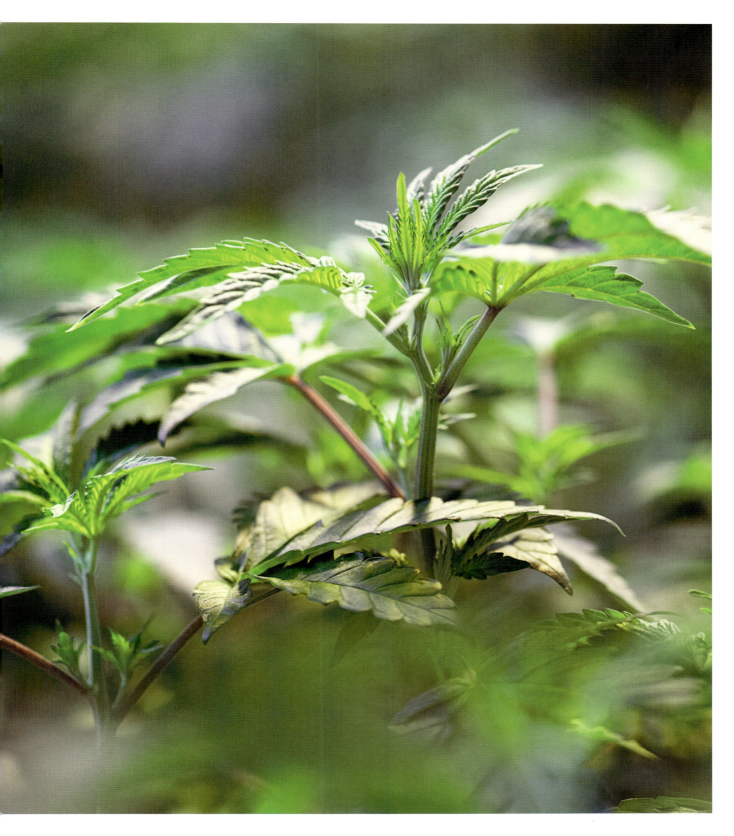

Decarboxylation:
Activating the Cannabinoids

To bring out the full flavor potential of herbs and spices, many cooks toast them before cooking. A similar principle applies to cannabis. When you expose this herb to even, gentle heat by toasting it in an oven, simmering it in a fat, or holding it to a flame, its flavor compounds and its THCA begins to convert to THC. Strong aromas erupt, creating an intricate palate of taste and scent and unlocking marijuana's psychoactive effects. This process is called decarboxylation (or "decarbing").

In order to get the most from your cannabis infusion, you first need to decarboxylate it. This process actives the THC and CBD in the plant. Without decarboxylation, cannabis is just a plain and simple herb. Thorough heating transforms its THCA from inactive organic material into the psychoactive THC we know and love.

Decarboxylation is a simple process with just a few steps:

🍁 Preheat oven to 240°F/116°C.

🍁 Break up cannabis flowers and buds into smaller pieces with your hands. We use 1 ounce, but you can elect to do more or less.

🍁 Place the cannabis in one layer on a rimmed baking sheet. Make sure the pan is the correct size: There should not be much empty space on the pan.

🍁 Bake the cannabis for forty minutes, stirring every fifteen minutes so that it cooks evenly.

🍁 When the cannabis is darker in color, a medium brown, and has dried out, remove the baking sheet and allow the cannabis to cool. It will be crumbly.

🍁 In a food processor, pulse the cannabis until it is coarsely ground (you don't want a superfine powder). Store it in an airtight container and use as needed to make extractions.

Making and Using Your Own Infusions

Once you become comfortable with making your own infusions, and understanding dosing and potency, you will be equipped to turn just about anything into an infused item. Caesar salad? Make infused croutons or infuse the dressing. T-bone steak? Top it with garlic canna-butter. Store-bought cookies? Decorate with an infused ganache or glaze.

Butter and olive oil that have been infused with cannabis are commonly referred to as canna-butter and canna-oil, and both are best kept in the refrigerator.

Knowing how to calibrate your infusions to dose them properly is key to consistent results. The THC potency can vary from strain to strain and between different harvests, sometimes wildly.

All recipes in this book are formulated with a consistent serving size of 5 milligrams of THC. The infusions are designed to result in a potency of 10 milligrams of THC per teaspoon using cannabis flower of 20 percent THC. Most strains on the shelves in Oregon are at least 20 percent THC, often up to 30 percent. How a bud can be 30 percent THC is beyond me, but that's what the results say. If you are lucky enough to live in a place with access to tested cannabis, you can refer to our guide to calibrate your infusion. Otherwise, you may need to test each batch of your infused butter yourself the old-fashioned way to assess your reaction to the potency.

THC can degrade at high heat—as a result, the recipes in this book all call for low to medium heat. Our motto when cooking with canna-butter or canna-oil is "low and slow."

When recipes require the use of an oven, the temperature never exceeds 340°F/171°C. In our recipe testing, we found that this was the highest temperature at which THC's potency could be preserved. To make sure you can replicate this in your own kitchen, you may wish to invest in an oven thermometer to calibrate the temperature of your oven.

Thorough mixing of the infused oil into the food is the most important step to ensure even distribution of THC throughout the dish. When the recipe calls for adding the canna-oil or canna-butter, be sure to mix thoroughly and scrape down the sides of the bowl, if needed, to incorporate every last bit.

Remember that each half teaspoon of canna-butter or canna-oil in the recipe equates to 5 milligrams of THC, our recommended serving size. Follow your own tolerance to determine whether you are able to consume a whole serving.

THC	CANNABIS
5%	76.5g
10%	38g
15%	25.5g
20%	19g
25%	15.25g
30%	12.8g

Testing for Potency Yourself

First things first: Make sure you're at home when you are tasting and testing. And plan to stay home. I recommend doing this in the evening, when you are less likely to need to run an errand for whatever reason. You can start by consuming a small amount of the infused oil or butter from a spoon. Because the butter or oil may be highly concentrated, start with $^1/_8$ teaspoon (or $^1/_{16}$ teaspoon, if you have it). This will also give you an idea of the taste you are going to be working with in your cooking and baking.

Personally, I do not enjoy the taste of infused butter or oil by itself. If you're the same way, why not do what I do and make pot brownies to test potency? If you make a batch of Triple Chocolate Starter Brownies (recipe found on page 166) with your butter or oil, just eat a tiny piece and wait a couple of hours to experience the effects. Although onset time varies, I suggest waiting four hours if you have to drive or operate heavy machinery. Perhaps you will get high, maybe you won't. That's okay; it's part of the plan.

Whatever you do, do not attempt to consume an entire brownie on the first night. You may want to eat more because they're hard to resist, but you must remain in control. If you require something sweet and delish, eat something non-infused. Sometimes I will make two batches of the brownies, one infused and one not. As long as you keep track of which is which, you can satisfy your munchies with great taste and no psychotropic results. Like snowflakes, no two people have the exact same tolerance. And from my experience, tolerance has nothing to do with gender or body mass. In my eyes, low tolerance is a blessing—you shouldn't feel a need to "prove" yourself by consuming too much.

By the next evening, if you feel like you want to increase your dose, allow yourself one whole brownie, containing 5 milligrams of THC. And then wait. And wait some more. Same rules apply: Stay home and relax; you are getting closer to your ideal edible dose. Once you have experienced an edible high, think of yourself as the

Goldilocks of marijuana: You need to determine whether your high is too low, too high, or just right. Another 2.5 milligrams of THC may do that, or another 25 milligrams of THC might. When it comes to cannabis, less is more. I'll say it again: Getting too high isn't fun. Adjust your dose as needed to find the dose that feels comfortable for you, and then stick with it.

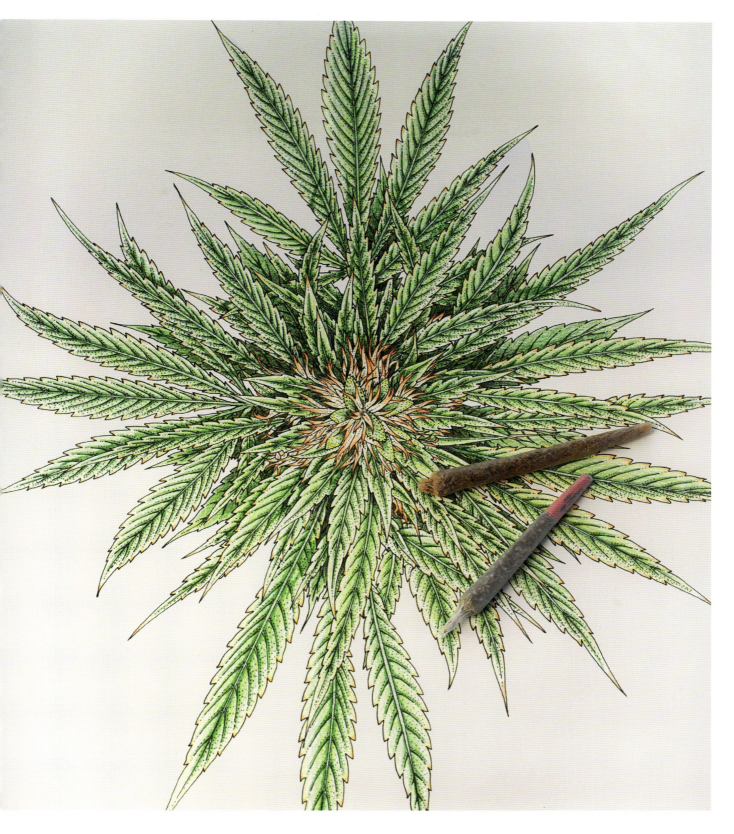

Infused Canna-Butter

Yield: 16 ounces infused canna-butter | Serving size: 1 teaspoon

When you're making canna-butter, the key thing to remember is "low and slow"—infusing the butter over low heat for several hours, never letting it boil, allows for full activation of the THC without scorching the herb. You can use any kind of unsalted butter you like, though we find that using high-quality butter provides a better taste. High-quality butter has less water, so you will get a higher yield.

Note that the finished butter will have a light green tinge to it because of the cannabis. Canna-butter will keep in the fridge for several weeks and in the freezer for up to six months. I vacuum-seal infused canna-butter to keep it airtight for prolonged storage. I have not noticed a significant degrading of potency or taste of canna-butter from the freezer when stored properly.

1 pound unsalted butter

Water, enough to fill the saucepan 1 to 2 inches

19 grams decarboxylated ground cannabis buds, or 38 grams decarboxylated dried, ground, and trimmed cannabis leaf

1. In a large saucepan, bring the butter and water to a simmer (just below a boil—the liquid will be active, with small bubbles consistently rising to the surface) over medium heat until the butter melts.

2. Whisk in the cannabis. Reduce the heat to low, and bring the mixture to a slow simmer (there will be very little movement in the liquid, with small bubbles occasionally rising to the surface). Do not let the mixture boil.

3. Cook for 3 hours, stirring every 30 minutes or so. Add additional warm water if needed (you don't want all the water to boil off).

4. While the butter cooks, line a strainer or sieve with cheesecloth, and place it over a large heat-safe glass bowl.

5. After 3 hours, pour the butter slowly through the cheesecloth and into the bowl. Press down on the cannabis with a spatula to extract all the butter. Fold the cheesecloth, and use the spatula to push any remaining canna-butter through the cloth and into the bowl. Discard the cheesecloth.

6. Cover the bowl with plastic wrap, and refrigerate it for at least 3 hours (overnight is better). The mixture will separate into solid butter and water.

7. Remove the butter from the fridge, slide a butter knife around the edges to remove the canna-butter from the bowl, and discard the water by pouring off.

8. Transfer the butter to a glass jar with a lid and store it in the fridge or freezer.

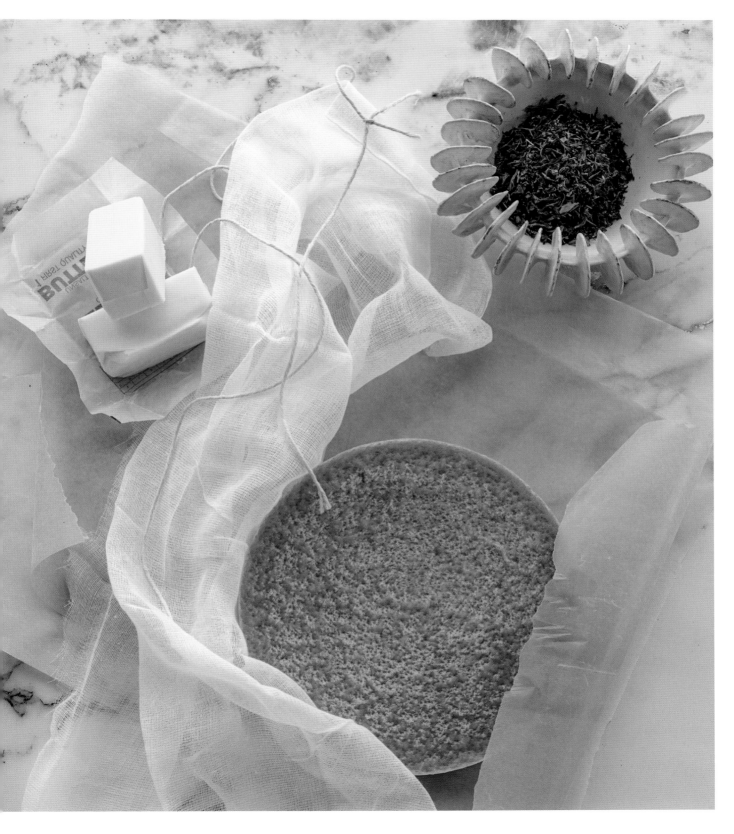

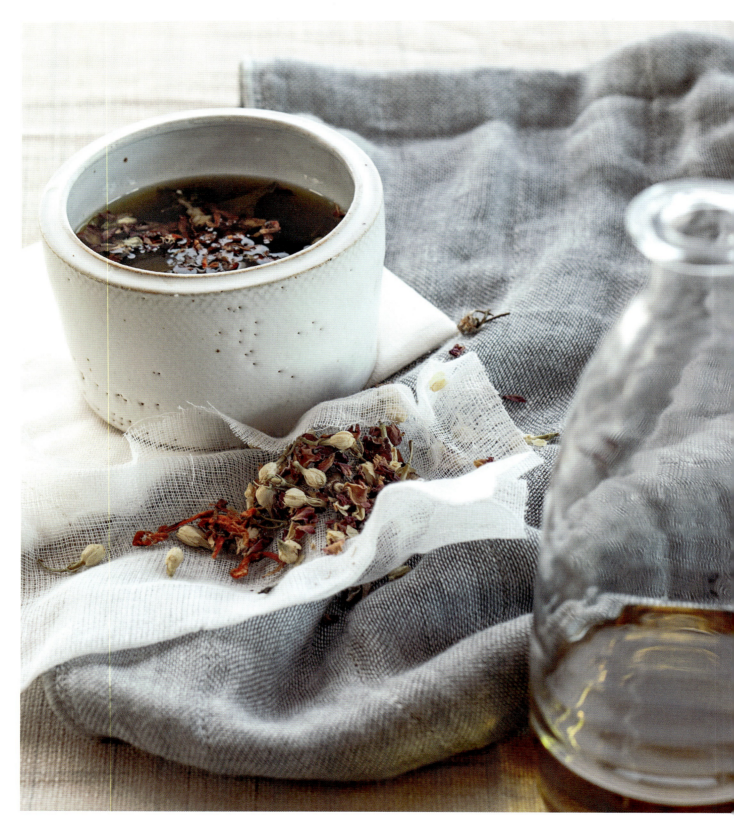

Infused Canna-Oil

Yield: 16 ounces infused canna-oil | Serving size: 1 teaspoon

---

You can use any type of cooking oil to make canna-oil, even a blend of two or more oils. The one exception is coconut oil, which, like butter, is solid at room temperature. To infuse coconut oil, you should follow the Infused Canna-Butter recipe. Other cooking oils require this technique. A good rule is to use the oils you already employ in your cooking, but some recipes in this book call specifically for canna–olive oil, canna–vegetable oil, or canna-coconut oil. In those cases, we chose a particular oil because it affects the taste of the final dish. Where it's not specified, you can use any type of canna-oil you have on hand. I often use a GMO-free canola oil, which is both tasteless and odorless.

Note that the finished canna-oil will have a green tinge to it because of the cannabis. Stored in a cool, dark place, canna-oil will easily keep for up to six months.

6 cups cooking oil of your choice (such as olive, avocado, peanut, coconut, grape-seed, sunflower, canola, or a mixture)

19 grams decarboxylated ground cannabis buds, or 38 grams decarboxylated dried, ground, and trimmed cannabis leaf

1. In the top of a double boiler, combine the cooking oil and the decarbed cannabis.

2. Do not let the bottom of the bowl touch the water. Cook the oil and the cannabis at a simmer for 3 hours. Stir every 30 minutes or so. Strain through several layers of cheesecloth. With the exception of coconut oil, this infusion will remain liquid, so do not add water. If using coconut oil, you can follow direction from the Infused Canna-Butter process.

Cannabis Flavor Profiles

For me, cooking with cannabis is akin to cooking with a new, occasionally dreadful-tasting herb. There are a lot of variables in the life of a cannabis plant, and the taste often varies, even if you use the same strain each time. For example, Blue Dream is a strain grown by hundreds of farmers, all doing their own thing. There will be differences in taste and potency due to the way the plant is grown and fertilized.

When cooking with cannabis, the more you know about the production of the plant, the better. Was it grown indoors or outdoors? Did the grower use pesticide-free, organic practices? Was the plant cured and properly stored?

Cannabis is a complicated plant, and there are multiple components that impact the consumer's experience of each strain. The terpene and cannabinoid profiles of the plant will inform its smell, taste, and psychological effects. There's a lot to learn, and if you are contemplating trying your hand with cannabis in the kitchen, knowing your terpenes will make you a better chef.

As you may remember from Chapter 2, terpenes are aromatic oils that give cannabis varieties their distinctive flavors and aromas. The potency levels for different strains of cannabis can be anywhere from 17 to 25 percent THC, and the terpene profiles can vary considerably. Not all variations will be huge, but it's certainly something to be aware of.

We just had an interesting experience in our bakery. We purchased cannabis flowers from a new source. We had smoked some of their herb and enjoyed it, so we were feeling optimistic about the results of our infusion and we made oil with ten pounds of flowers. The result was kind of bizarre in that the batch of oil that we made was absolutely incompatible with the flavor profile of our Peanut Butter Blondies. It made for an absolutely dreadful taste. That had never happened before. The same oil infused several of our other products with no negative results. Something unpleasant happened when the peanut butter met this particular oil. We had to throw out the whole batch of 2,500 blondies. That experience was painful, but it served to remind us that there are potential changes every time you buy or procure a new batch of cannabis, and it is important to taste test with every new flavor combination. There is more consistency when you buy the same strain—say, Blue Dream—from the same farm every time, but even then, you can expect slight discrepancies. It definitely keeps us on our toes.

I've found that there are a couple of terpenes that seem to always work with the types of food that I enjoy cooking. They are limonene and myrcene. Limonene is citrusy and fresh, and I love to use that strain for salads, soups, and desserts. Myrcene is the most common terpene, and I like to use it in Asian cooking and infusing tropical desserts with coconut and mango. Pinene is my least favorite terpene to cook with. It's piney (surprise) and tastes bitter to me. I have used it in stuffed mushrooms and earthy stews with some success, but I personally don't like smoking it or tasting it. But that should not dissuade you from experimenting with different strains. If you are making an oil or butter with a fairly potent strain, the amount you would use to infuse will be minimal. A teaspoon of the infused oil will not necessarily make or break your recipe; and it is likely to be potent enough to do the job.

Terpene Flavor Pairings

BETACARYOPHELLENE

Taste: Sharp, pepper, rosemary, cloves

Found in: cloves, hops, rosemary

Effects: pain relief, inflammation relief

Strains: Death Star, Candyland, Girl Scout Cookie (GSC)

Pairs well with: grilled meats, stir fry, eggs, cheese,
spaghetti carbonara, chocolate chip cookies with coarse salt

D-LIMONENE

Taste: citrusy, fresh

Found in: citrus fruit

Effects: antianxiety, antidepression, stress relief

Strains: Lemon Haze, Hindu Kush, Dirty Girl

Pairs well with: orange smoothies, lemon curd tarts,
grapefruit arugula salad, poke

LINALOOL

Taste: robust, floral, spicy

Found in: lavender, mint

Effects: anticonvulsant, antianxiety, anti-nausea

Strains: Granddaddy Purple, LA Confidential, Lavender, Bubba Kush

Pairs well with: seafood, desserts, lavender lemonade

MYRCENE

Taste: spicy, herbal, mango

Found in: thyme, parsley, bay leaf, mango

Effects: sedating, analgesic

Strains: Pure Kush, Himalayan Gold, Jack Herer

Pairs well with: mango salsa, lemongrass grilled chicken, rosemary potatoes

PINENE

Taste: pine-scented bouquet

Found in: pine trees, basil, rosemary, parsley

Effects: opens airways in lungs, enhances memory, alert, attentive, counteracts paranoia

Strains: White Widow, Trainwreck, 9 Pound Hammer, Blue Dream

Pairs well with: stuffed mushrooms, hearty stews, robust flavors

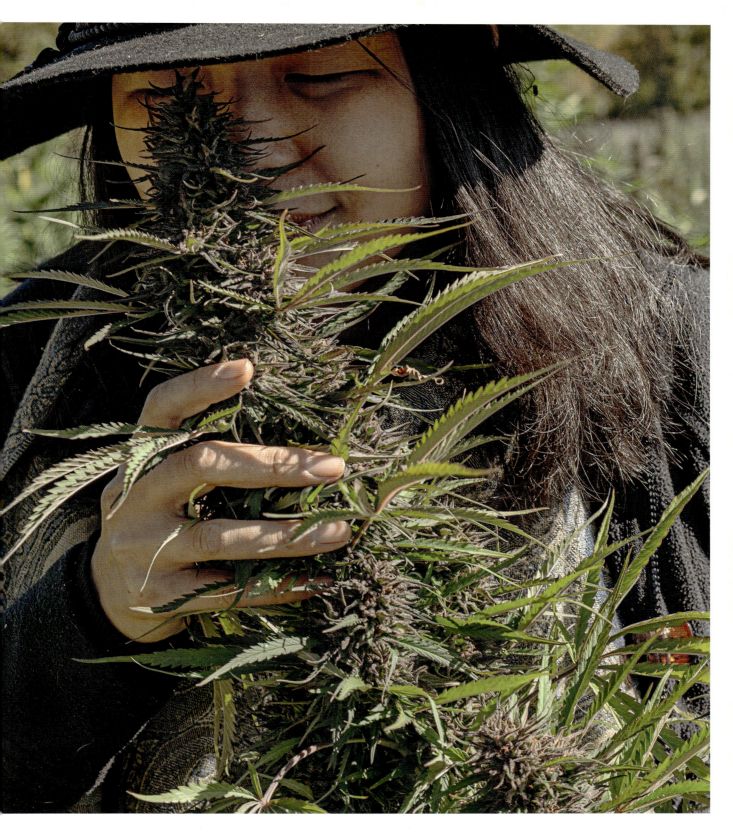

Triple Chocolate Starter Brownies

Yield: 12 brownies | Serving: 1 brownie | THC: 5 milligrams per serving

Earlier I mentioned baking brownies as a home cannabis potency test. And who doesn't want a brownie recipe?

I think the brownie continues to be *the* cannabis dessert and many people's first experience with cannabis edibles. Too often the potency is unknown or too high, and the experience can be an unpleasant introduction to edibles. This recipe is formulated to produce a pleasant serving of 5 milligrams of THC per brownie.

Chocolate and cannabis are perfect pairings, and an infused brownie is always a wonderful, welcoming place to start. These brownies need no embellishing; however, if you are feeling fancy, top a square with ice cream and fudge sauce or fresh berries and whipped cream.

Baking spray

4 ounces semisweet chocolate, chopped

¾ cup all-purpose flour

¼ cup cocoa powder

1 teaspoon salt

10 tablespoons unsalted butter

2 tablespoons canna-butter

1¼ cups granulated sugar

2 large eggs

1 tablespoon vanilla extract

4 ounces semisweet chocolate chips

1. Heat oven to 340°F/171°C. Spray and line an 8-by-8-inch baking pan with parchment paper.

2. In a microwave-safe bowl, melt chopped chocolate at 30-second intervals. Test to see if the chocolate is melted by stirring with a spoon; sometimes it isn't obvious to the eye.

3. In a small bowl, combine the flour, cocoa powder, and salt.

4. In a large bowl, beat the butters and sugar until light and fluffy, 5–7 minutes. Add the eggs and the vanilla, and beat for an additional 5 minutes.

5. Beat in the melted chocolate. Gently fold the dry ingredients into the butter/sugar mixture. Don't overmix! You can tell when it's ready by seeing an absence of flour lumps—you only want to mix until you don't see any.

6. Add the chocolate chips, and fold to combine. Bake for 18–22 minutes. Let cool, and cut into 12 even squares, if you wish.

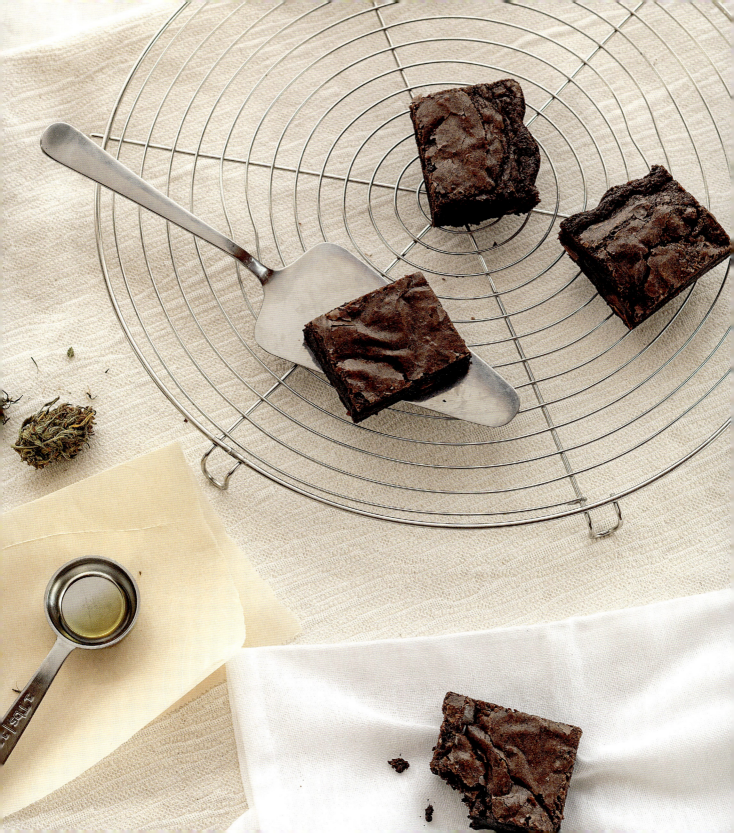

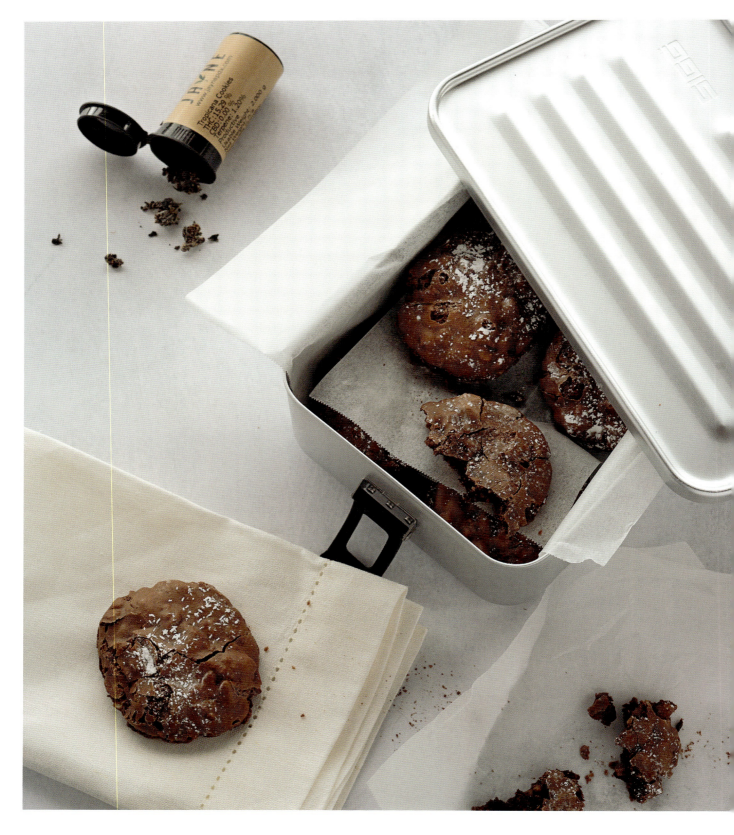

Chocolate Crinkle Cookies

Yield: 18 cookies | Servings: 18 (1 cookie per serving)

THC: 5 milligrams per serving

You know that little voice in your head that says, "Put down the cookies, Laurie, and back away slowly"? Well, to that little voice I say, "You don't own me," and continue devouring these delicious cookies. They're called "Crinkle Cookies" because the sugar coating caramelizes during the baking process, which gives them a delightful crunch.

½ cup granulated sugar

3 tablespoons melted canna-butter or canna-oil

1 ounce unsweetened chocolate, melted and cooled

1 teaspoon vanilla extract

1 large egg, lightly beaten

½ cup all-purpose flour

½ teaspoon baking powder

Healthy pinch of salt

½ cup confectioners' sugar

1. Prepare cookie sheets with parchment. Set aside.

2. In a large bowl, beat the sugar, canna-butter or canna-oil, chocolate, and vanilla. Beat in the egg.

3. In another bowl, combine the flour, baking powder, and salt. Add the dry ingredients to the chocolate mixture, and beat to combine. Chill for several hours.

4. Heat oven to 340°F/171°C. Place confectioners' sugar in a bowl. Form the batter into 1-inch balls and roll in the sugar. Place the balls 2 inches apart on prepared cookie sheets. Bake for 9–11 minutes. Cool on a wire rack.

Deep Dark Chocolate Almond Clusters

Yield: 36 clusters | Servings: 18 (2 clusters per serving)

THC: 5 milligrams per serving

This combination of flavors is one of my favorites. Get the darkest chocolate you can, and make sure the almonds are crunchy. Much of this recipe is good for you, and it tastes so good you will never want to stop. But you must; in life we all do things we don't want to do.

Be careful not to let any water get in the bowl with the melting chocolate. The chocolate will seize, and nothing good will happen. It will require a redo, and we certainly don't want that to happen.

1½ cups dark chocolate chips or melts (vegan chips or even carob would work well here)

3 tablespoons canna–coconut oil

1 cup well-roasted almonds

⅓ cup chopped dried cherries

Fleur de Sel, optional

1. In a double boiler, heat the chocolate along with the canna–coconut oil.

2. When fully melted, remove from heat. Stir in the almonds and cherries.

3. Place parchment paper on your work surface. Drop 1 tablespoon of the chocolate mixture onto the paper. Sprinkle with a pinch of salt if you are so inclined.

4. Allow to set and cool completely, at least 60 minutes.

5. Store in a labeled, airtight container.

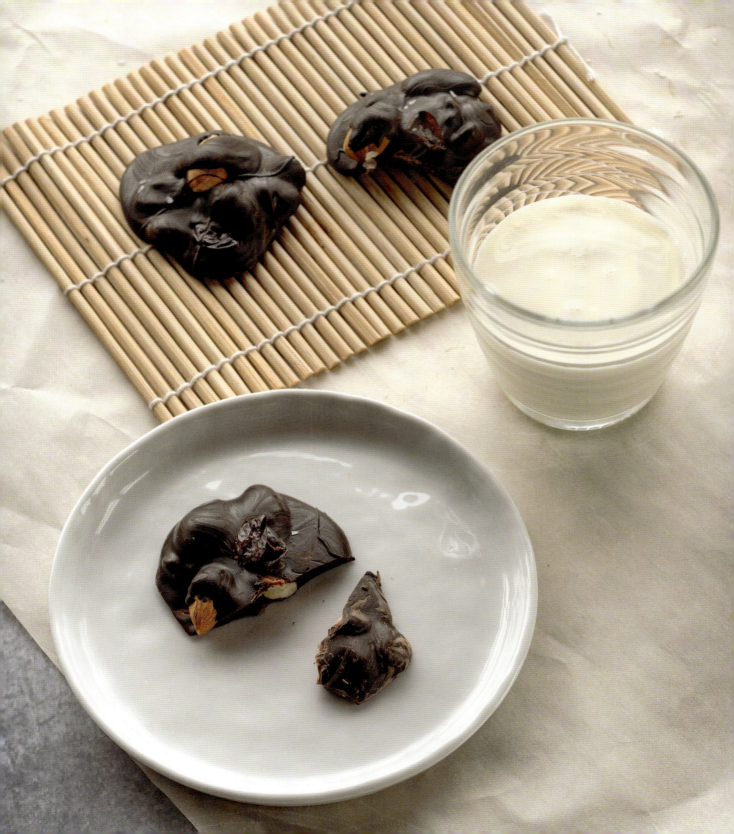

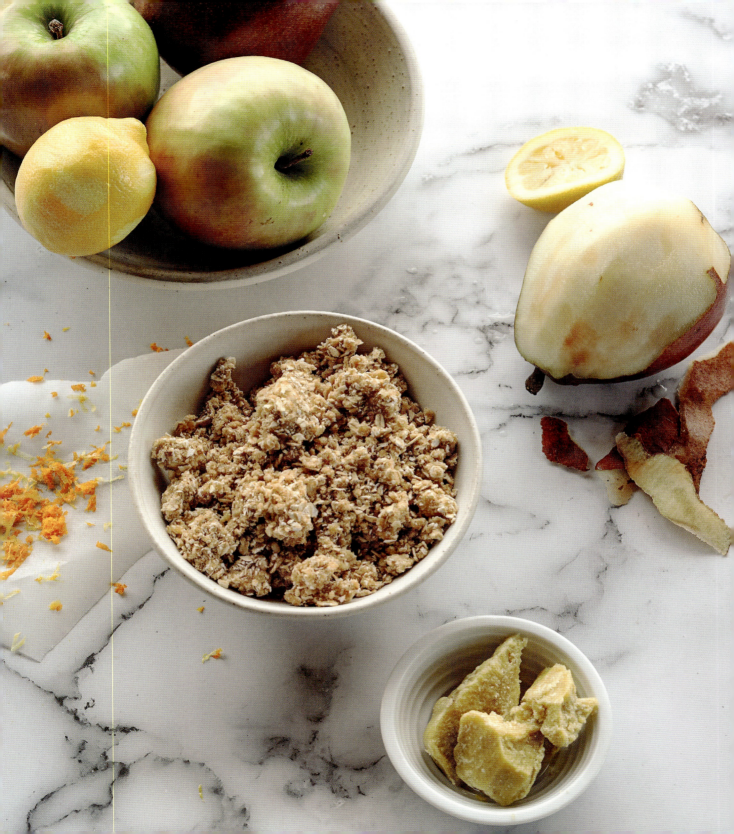

Seasonal Fruit and Cannabis Crumble

Yield: 9 pieces | Servings: 9 (1 piece per serving) | THC: 5 milligrams per serving

When I bake this dish, I always double the amount of topping and keep it in the freezer for dessert emergencies. The fruit can be frozen when you bake the crumble, so things can come together pretty quickly. Your home will be perfumed with irresistible aromas, and you may need to be restrained while giving the dessert thirty minutes after it is done baking to become what it is meant to be. Maybe smoke a joint and chillax while you wait. In the summer months, adjust the fruit. I'm a firm believer in the magic between peaches and blueberries. And crystalized ginger.

FRUIT MIXTURE

Baking spray

2 pounds ripe pears, peeled and sliced (I like Bosc)

2 pounds Granny Smith apples, peeled and sliced

8 ounces dates, chopped

1 teaspoon fresh lemon zest

1 teaspoon fresh orange zest

4 tablespoons orange juice concentrate

½ cup light brown sugar, packed

¼ cup all-purpose flour

1 teaspoon cinnamon

¼ teaspoon cardamom

¼ teaspoon nutmeg

Pinch of salt

CRUMBLE

1½ cups all-purpose flour

1 cup regular oats

¾ cup light brown sugar, packed

¾ cup granulated sugar

½ teaspoon salt

12 tablespoons unsalted butter

1½ tablespoons canna-butter

1. Heat oven to 325°F/163°C. Spray a large baking dish and set aside. In a large bowl, combine the pears, apples, dates, zests, juice concentrate, brown sugar, flour, cinnamon, nutmeg, and salt.

2. Place the fruit mixture in the large prepared dish.

3. In another large bowl, combine the flour, oats, brown sugar, white sugar, salt, and butters. Using your (clean) hands, mix the topping ingredients until crumbly. It's okay if there are still bits of butter showing.

4. Sprinkle the topping over the fruit mixture. Bake for 1 hour, until the crumble is golden brown and the juices are bubbling. Serve warm, perhaps with a scoop of ice cream on top.

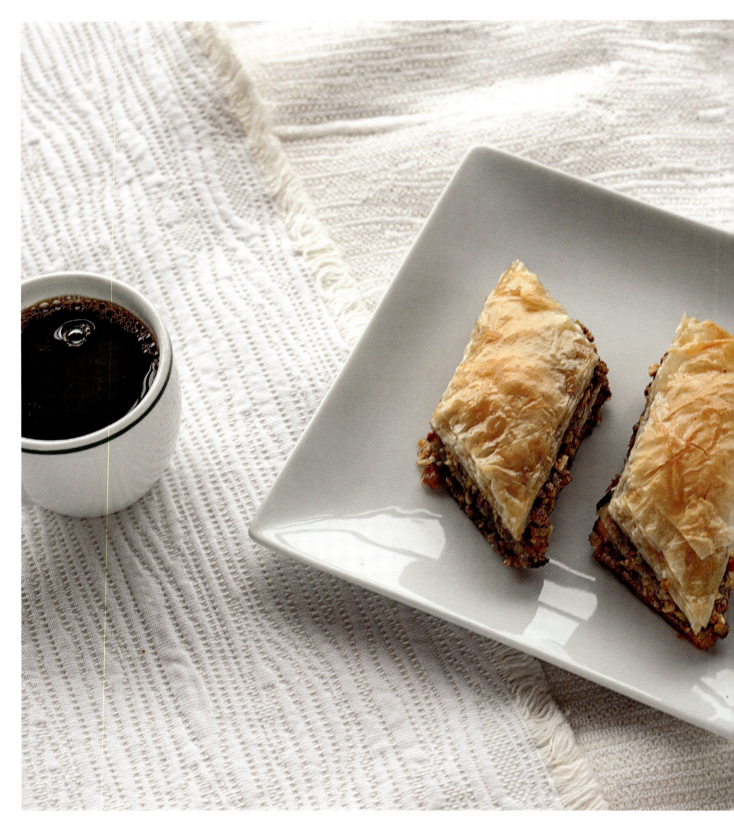

Pistachio and Rose Baklava

Yield: 30 pieces | Servings: 30 (1 piece per serving)

THC: 5 milligrams per serving

———————

Sometimes I really want something crunchy to eat. But I don't always eat fried chicken, or egg rolls, or toast. I want something sweet and crunchy; something to take the edge off. I turn to my baklava recipe to achieve this, because it's the perfect treat to nosh on when I feel like washing my hands later.

1 pound of pistachios, lightly toasted

1 (16-ounce) package phyllo dough

5 tablespoons canna-butter, melted

11 tablespoons unsalted butter, melted

1 cup granulated sugar

1 cup water

1 teaspoon vanilla extract

½ cup honey

1 tablespoon rose water

1. Heat oven to 340°F/171°C. Butter the bottom and sides of a 9-by-13-inch baking pan. In a food processor, chop the pistachios into a medium-fine texture. In a small bowl, combine both butters and mix well.

2. Unroll the phyllo dough. Cover the phyllo with a lightly dampened cloth to keep from drying out as you work. Place two sheets of dough in the pan, and brush with the butter. Place another sheet of dough on top, and repeat with individual sheets of phyllo until you have layered 12 sheets.

3. When 12 layers are reached, sprinkle the chopped nuts on top. From here, continue in layering pattern, adding the nuts with the butter in between each layer of dough. The top layers should be near 6–8 sheets high.

4. Using a sharp knife, cut to the bottom of the pan into diamond or square shapes. Bake for about 50 minutes, until baklava is golden and crisp.

5. While the baklava is baking is the ideal time to make the sauce! Boil sugar and water until sugar is melted. Add vanilla, honey, and rose water. Simmer slowly for about 45 minutes. Remove baklava from oven and immediately pour sauce over it. Let cool, and then enjoy.

Lemon Curd on Toasted Baguette

Yield: 12 slices of baguette topped with infused lemon curd
Servings: 12 (1 slice per serving) | THC: 5 milligrams per serving

This beautiful dessert turned me into a lemon lover. Everything about it is lovely: It's tart and sweet, smooth and crunchy, simple and beautiful. If fresh berries are not in season, garnish the curd with lightly toasted sliced almonds and toasted coconut flakes. Drizzle with chocolate only if you feel like a badass!

2 large lemons, zested and juiced (a generous half cup)

1 cup granulated sugar

5 egg yolks, lightly beaten

6 tablespoons unsalted butter, cut in pieces

2 tablespoons canna-butter, cut in pieces

½ teaspoon vanilla extract

Pinch of salt

12 slices baguette, toasted

1 cup fresh berries, sliced if large

⅓ cup flaked coconut

1. In a medium bowl, combine the zest and sugar. Mash them together with a wooden spoon or potato masher.

2. In a medium saucepan, combine the zest-and-sugar mixture, lemon juice, yolks, and butters. Stir to mix well. Cook the mixture over low/medium heat, stirring frequently, until the butters are melted and the mixture thickens, about 12–15 minutes. Remove from heat and place in a bowl. Stir in the vanilla and salt.

3. The mixture will continue to thicken as it cools. Place plastic wrap against the curd and chill for at least 2 hours.

4. Spread the curd over the toasted bread. Top with berries and flaked coconut.

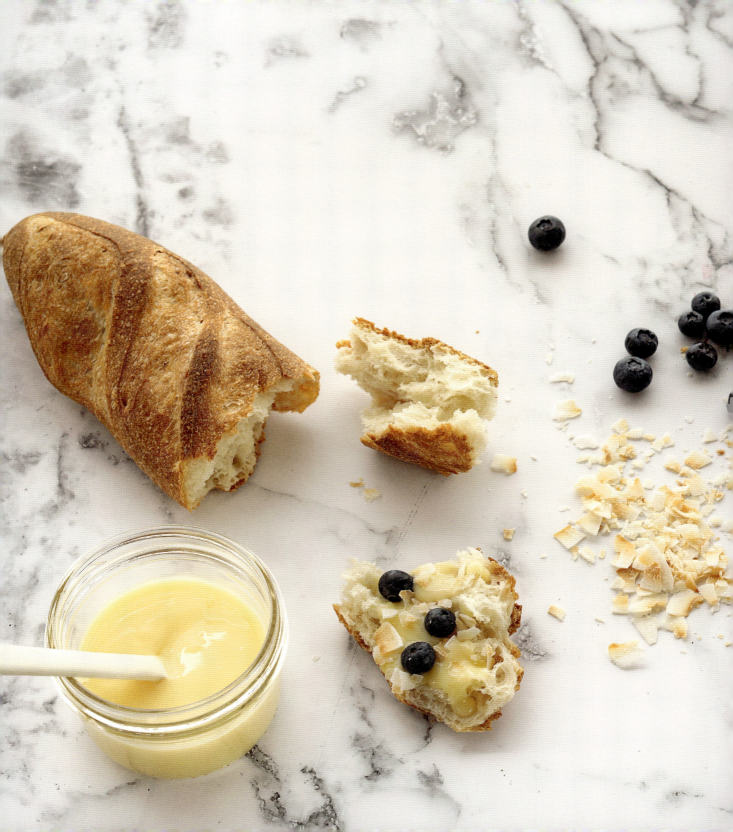

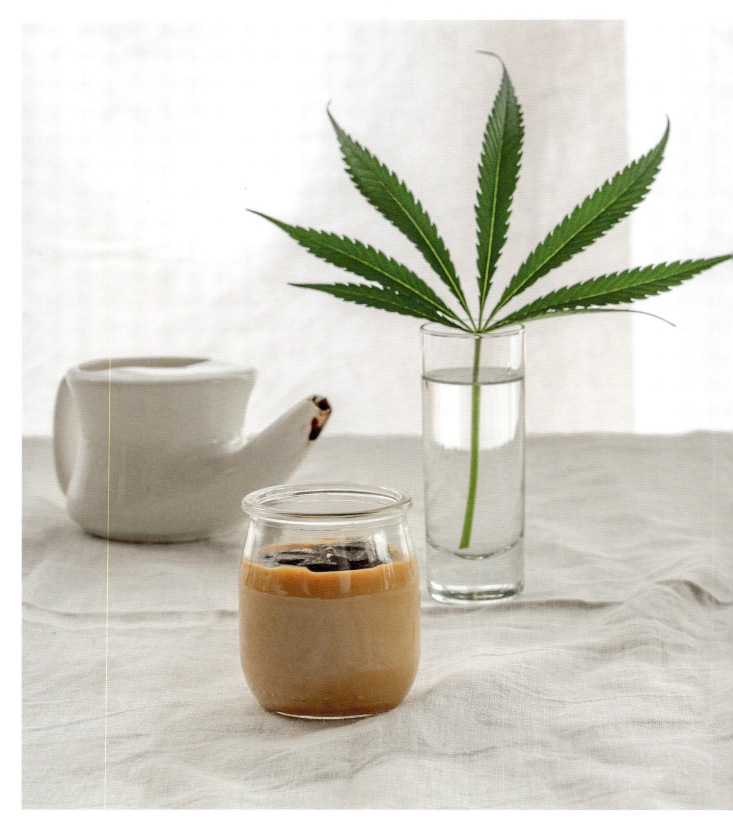

Butterscotch Budino

Yield: 4 Budinos | Servings: 4 (1 Budino per serving)

THC: 5 milligrams per serving

I love a Budino. It's like that song "I Love a Piano" by Irving Berlin. Budinos are a smooth, creamy pudding that has become popular in restaurants over the last few years. Maybe it's the richness created by the half-and-half (some chefs use heavy cream, too).

½ cup dark brown sugar, packed

2 tablespoons, plus 2 teaspoons cornstarch

⅛ teaspoon salt

2 cups half-and-half

2 lightly beaten egg yolks

2 teaspoons canna-butter

2 teaspoons vanilla extract

4 tablespoons heavy cream

½ cup semisweet chocolate chips

1. In a small saucepan, combine the brown sugar, cornstarch, and salt. Add the half-and-half and yolks, and stir until smooth.

2. Cook over low/medium heat until mixture comes to a simmer. Stir constantly for 1–2 minutes, until the mixture thickens.

3. Remove the saucepan from the heat, and add the butter and vanilla. Allow to cool to room temperature, stirring a couple of times, then pour into individual cups before chilling for 3–4 hours.

4. In a small microwave-safe dish, heat the cream for 30 seconds. Add the chocolate chips, and stir until melted and smooth. Place 1 tablespoon of this chocolate mixture on the top of each budino cup.

Chocolate Chess Pie

Yield: 8 slices | Servings: 8 (1 slice per serving) | THC: 5 milligrams per serving

If you have never had a chess pie, now is the time. The velvety texture, the deep rich flavor, the cannabis, you may be hooked—but in a good way. It's easy to make, and you can always take a shortcut and buy a premade crust. There are pretty good ones out there. Once I made the filling with a graham cracker crust and it rocked. Slightly s'mores-ish.

CRUST
Baking spray

1¼ cups all-purpose flour

1 tablespoon granulated sugar

½ teaspoon salt

8 tablespoons chopped, cold, unsalted butter

2–4 tablespoons ice water

2 cups pie weights or dried beans

FILLING
13 tablespoons unsalted butter

3 tablespoons canna-butter

4 ounces good-quality semisweet chocolate

2 tablespoons good-quality cocoa powder

2 cups granulated sugar

4 large eggs, lightly beaten

4 teaspoons vanilla extract

Pinch of salt

WHIPPED TOPPING
1 cup heavy cream, very cold

2 teaspoons vanilla extract

3 tablespoons confectioners' sugar

1 tablespoon good-quality cocoa powder

1. Spray a deep 9-inch pie plate and set aside.

2. In a food processor, combine the flour, sugar, and salt. Pulse to combine. Add the butter and pulse again, adding 1 teaspoon of ice water at a time until the dough clumps together. Gather the dough, form it into a disc, wrap it in parchment, and chill for a minimum of 45 minutes.

3. Remove the dough and place on a well-floured work surface. Roll the dough out to an 11–12-inch circle. Gently lift the crust and place in the prepared pie pan; there should be at least an inch overhang. Fold the excess crust under itself. Press together, and press the crust edge all around with the tines of a fork. Chill the crust for 15 minutes.

4. Heat oven to 400°F/204°C.

5. Remove the crust from the fridge and place a piece of parchment paper or foil on the crust. Cover the whole thing. Place the weights or beans on the foil or parchment. Bake the crust for 15 minutes. Carefully remove the foil with the weights, and place the crust back in the oven for 5–7 minutes, or until golden brown.

6. To make the filling, heat the uninfused and infused butters, chocolate, and cocoa powder in a medium microwavable bowl at half power, in 30-second intervals, stirring after each. Allow to cool.

7. In a medium bowl, beat the sugar, eggs, vanilla, and salt. Add to the chocolate mixture. Reduce the heat to 340°F/171°C.

8. Pour the mixture into the pie shell and bake for 30–35 minutes, until the edges are set and the center is just a touch jiggly. Jiggly is a weird yet fun word.

9. For the whipped topping, beat the heavy cream, vanilla, sugar, and cocoa powder on medium speed in a medium bowl until medium peaks form, 2–3 minutes.

10. Cool the pie, cut into 8 even slices, and serve with the whipped cream (wait to have a second piece when the cannabis kicks in).

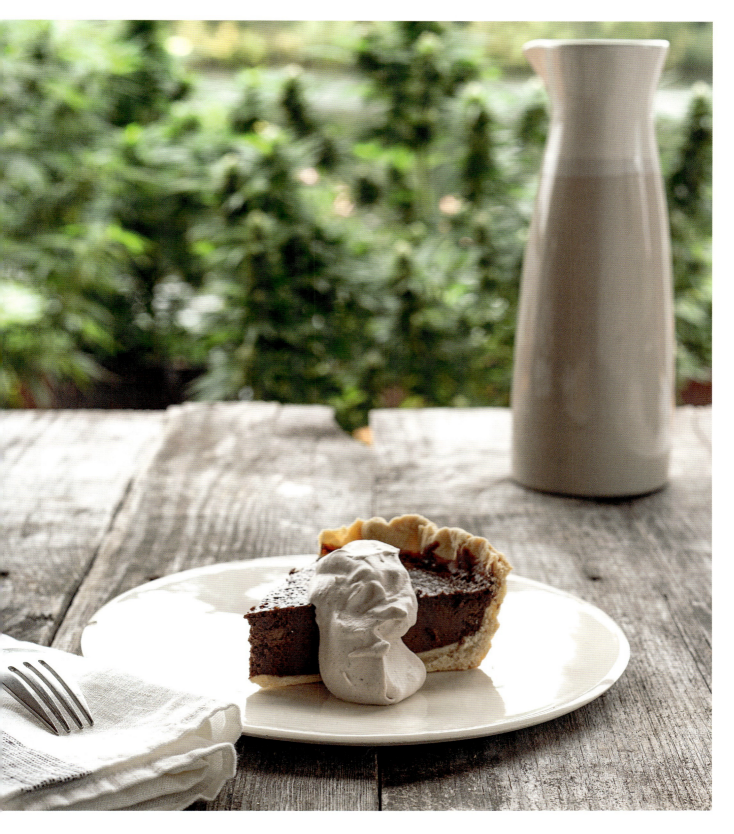

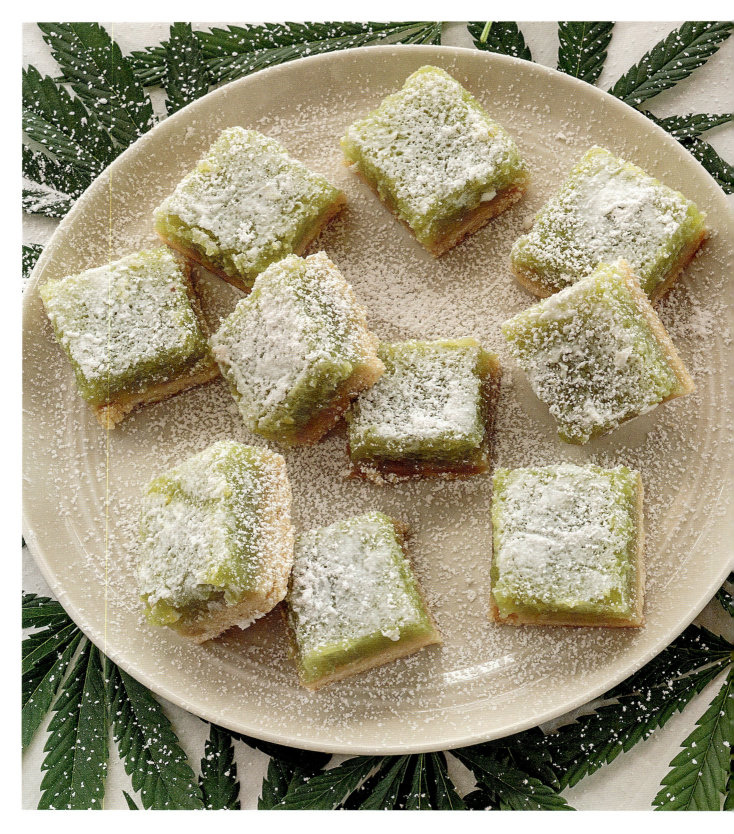

Double Citrus Bars

Yield: 12 citrus bars | Servings: 12 (1 piece per serving)

THC: 5 milligrams per serving

It's like a lemon bar, but better. These goodies have a complementing mix of lemons as well as limes, and the sweetness is adjustable to your liking. The creaminess from the, well, cream is also a major player in making this recipe a family favorite.

CRUST

Baking spray

2 cups all-purpose flour

½ cup granulated sugar

¼ teaspoon salt

6 tablespoons cold unsalted butter

2 tablespoons cold canna-butter

LEMON-LIME FILLING

4 large eggs, lightly beaten

1½ cups granulated sugar

⅓ cup half-and-half

3 tablespoons all-purpose flour

1 teaspoon lemon zest

⅓ cup lemon juice

1 teaspoon lime zest

⅓ cup lime juice

1 drop green food coloring, optional

Confectioners' sugar for topping

Extra lemon and lime zest for topping

CRUST

1. Spray a 9-by-13-inch baking pan with baking spray. Cover the bottom with parchment paper.

2. Heat oven to 325°F/163°C. In a large bowl, combine the flour, sugar, and salt. Whisk to combine.

3. Add the butters, and mix with your fingers to form a mixture that resembles oatmeal. Press into the bottom of the prepared pan. Bake in the oven for 15 minutes; it will ideally be a light golden brown when finished.

FILLING

1. In a large bowl, combine the eggs, sugar, half-and-half, flour, lemon zest, lemon juice, lime zest, lime juice, and food coloring, if using.

2. Pour the mixture on top of the baked crust. Bake at 340°F/171°C until the filling is set, about 15–20 minutes. Allow to cool fully before cutting into 12 servings. If desired, dust with confectioners' sugar and grated zest.

White Chocolate Granola Clusters

Yield: 24 clusters | Serving: 2 clusters

THC: 5 milligrams per serving (60 milligrams total)

The question I get asked most often—other than "Do you have any weed?"—is whether I like the taste of cannabis in the food I cook. It can be tricky to pair cannabis with some food, since it often requires extra spicing to get the correct flavors. White chocolate, granola, and cannabis are a great taste trio. It gets me every time.

2 cups white chocolate chips

2 tablespoons coconut oil

2 tablespoons infused coconut oil

1 cup granola

1 cup semisweet chocolate chips

1. Place a 24-cup mini muffin tin on your work surface and place a liner in each cup.

2. In a double boiler over low heat, melt the white chocolate with the coconut oil and the infused coconut oil. When fully melted, remove from heat. Using a spoon, drop the melted chocolate into the muffin tin, creating 24 cluster bases. Sprinkle each base with 1 teaspoon of the granola while the chocolate is still warm.

3. In a double boiler, melt the semisweet chocolate. When fully melted, spoon the chocolate over the white chocolate clusters, filling the muffin tin $2/3$ of the way up the paper liner. Top each cluster with another heaping teaspoon of granola. Allow to set before moving or eating, about 30 minutes.

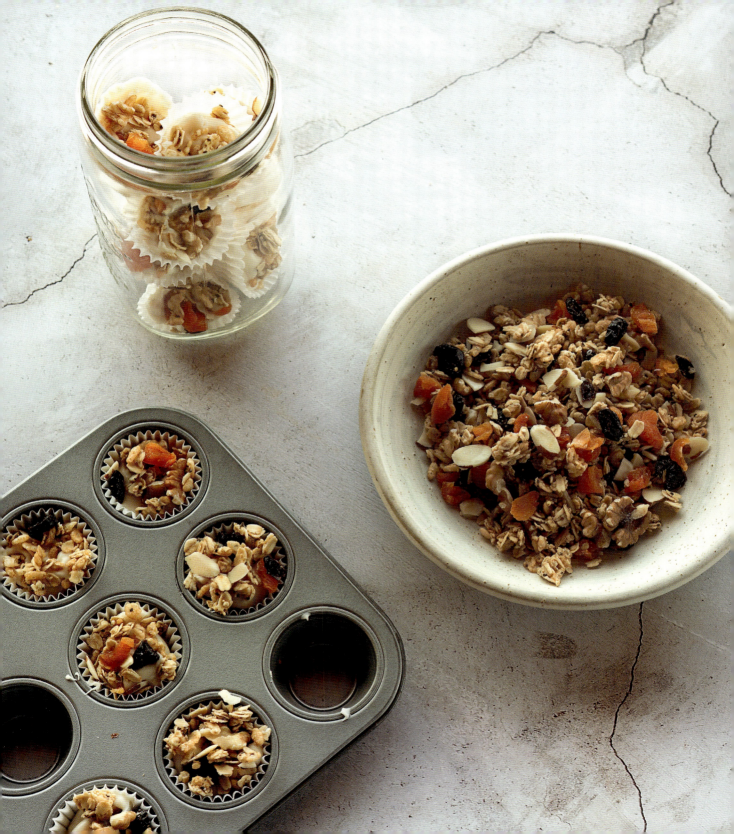

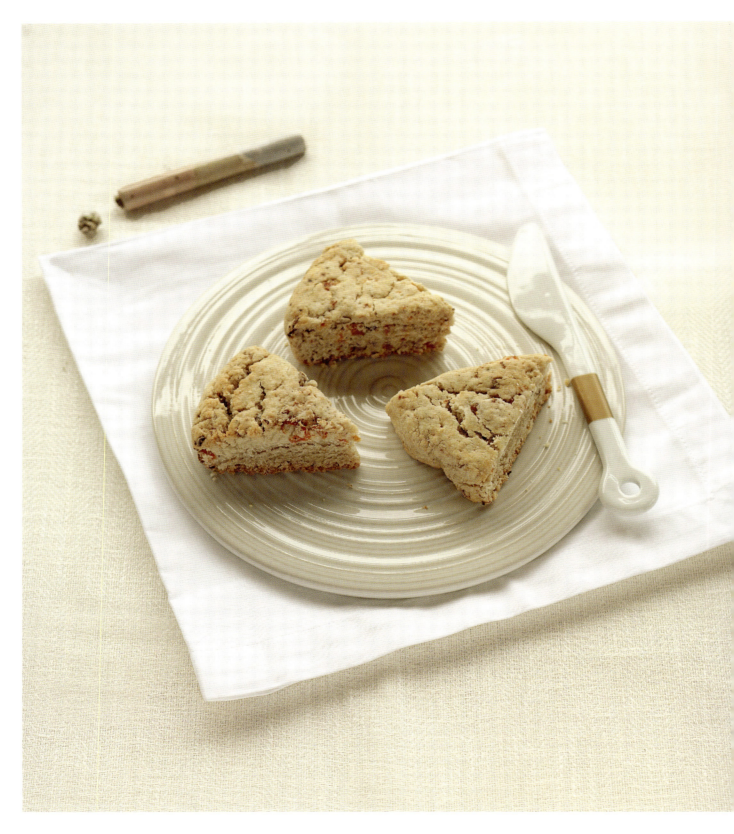

Apricot Orange Mini Scones

Yield: 16 scones | Serving: 1 scone | THC: 5 milligrams per serving

For several years I have been making scones for an English friend. She'll give my scones a grade, which sounds much harsher than it is. I've gotten better. My last scone delivery got me an 8.9.

3 cups all-purpose flour

1 tablespoon baking powder

¼ teaspoon salt

⅓ cup granulated sugar, plus more for garnish

1 tablespoon orange zest

5 tablespoons butter, cold and cubed

3 tablespoons canna-butter, cold and cubed

¾ cup milk, plus more for brushing on scones

2 large eggs, lightly beaten

1 teaspoon vanilla

¼ teaspoon orange extract

½ cup chopped dried apricots

½ cup chopped pecans

1. Heat the oven to 340°F/171°C.

2. Line a large baking sheet with parchment paper and set aside.

3. In a large bowl, combine the flour, baking powder, and salt.

4. In a small bowl, combine the sugar and orange zest. Mix into the flour mixture until evenly distributed.

5. Add the chunks of cold butter and canna-butter to the flour mixture. Cut in the butter using a pastry blender or your clean hands. I like to use my hands so that I can feel when I have the right texture. Mix until you have pea-size chunks of butter.

6. In a medium bowl, combine the milk, eggs, and vanilla. Mix with the dry ingredients until moist. Add the apricots and pecans, and gently mix into the dough. Transfer the dough to a work surface lightly dusted with flour. Knead gently until the dough comes together.

7. Shape the dough into two small circles, each about 7 inches. Cut each dough circle into 8 wedges and place the wedges on the prepared baking sheet. Don't worry if the wedges are not exactly the same size. Brush each scone with milk and sprinkle with sugar. Bake for 13–15 minutes, or until the scones are light golden brown. Remove from the oven and allow to cool.

Dipped Mango

Yield: 12 pieces | Serving: 2 pieces

THC: 5 milligrams per serving (30 milligrams total)

Since I rarely find a ripe mango, these dried slices are an awesome substitute. There is some serious talk in the cannabis world about how the terpene myrcene, which occurs naturally in mangoes, works with the myrcene in the cannabis to create an intensified high. Whether that's true or not, when you taste this combination of mango, chocolate, and almonds, you will be thrilled. This is also great dipped in coconut instead of almonds.

1 cup dark chocolate chips

1 tablespoon infused coconut oil

12 large pieces dried mango

¼ cup toasted almond slivers

1. Line a baking sheet with parchment.

2. In a small microwave-safe bowl, heat the chocolate for 30 seconds. Check and stir to see if it is melted. Sometimes chips have melted but you can't tell. If you need more heating time, microwave at 15-second intervals. Stir in the infused coconut oil.

3. Dip each mango piece into the melted chocolate and place on the parchment. Sprinkle with the almonds.

4. Allow the chocolate to set, at least 30 minutes.

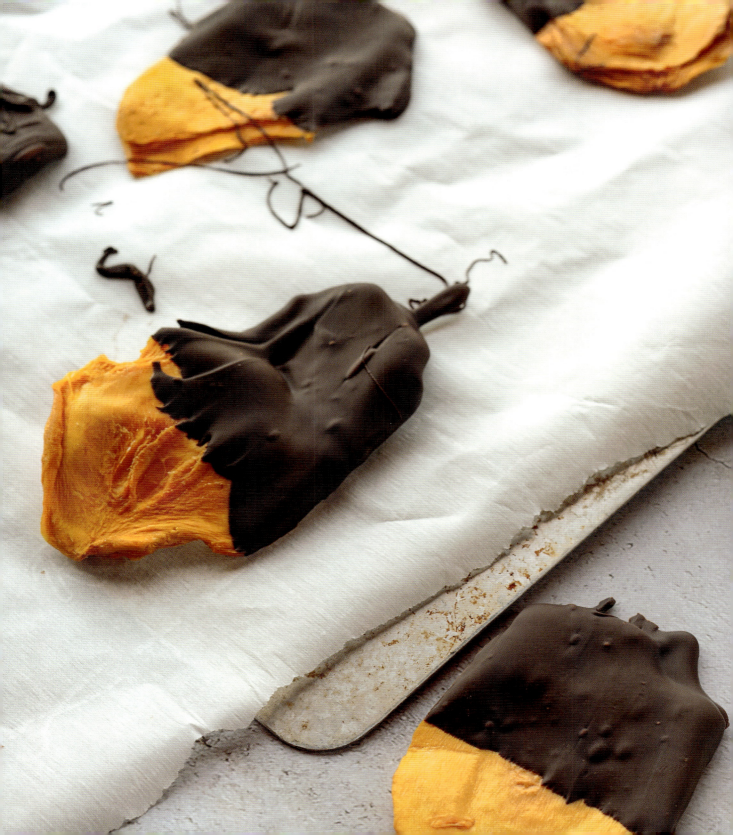

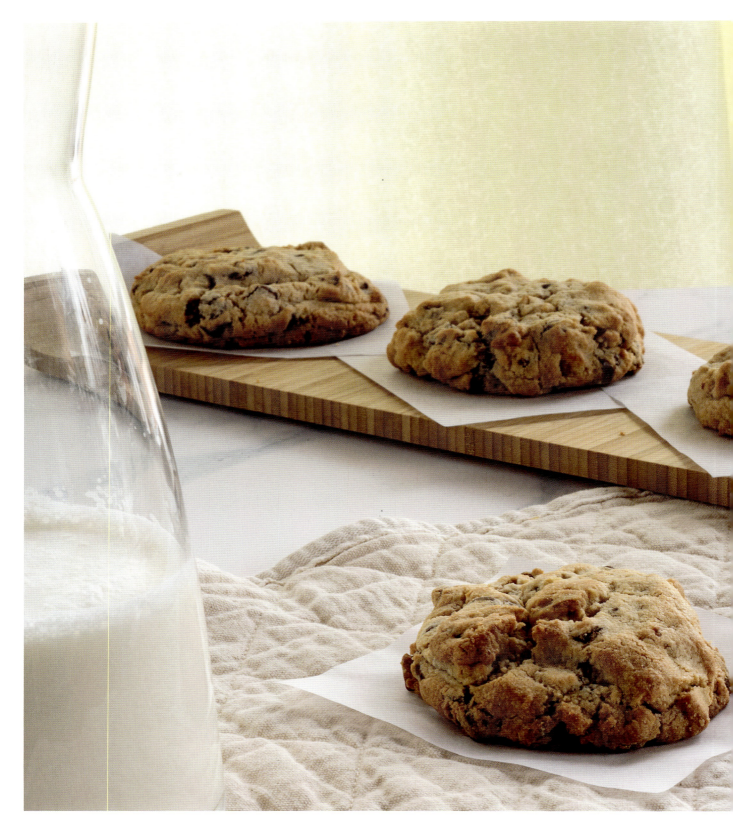

Big, Very Big, Chocolate Chip Cookies

Yield: 8 cookies | Serving: 1 cookie
THC: 5 milligrams per serving (40 milligrams total)

My friend Freddi told me about some cookies from Levain, a bakery in New York City. They sounded so good that I decided to spend a fortune and have them delivered to Oregon. Yes, they are great. This homemade version is very good as well, and instead of flying them across the country, I get to eat them 20 minutes after they come out of the oven.

6½ tablespoons butter, softened

4 teaspoons canna-butter, softened

¾ cup firmly packed light brown sugar

½ cup granulated sugar

2 large eggs, room temperature

2 teaspoons vanilla paste

1 cup cake flour

1½ cups all-purpose flour

1 teaspoon baking powder

1 teaspoon baking soda

½ teaspoon sea salt

4 cups semisweet chocolate chips

1. Heat the oven to 340°F/171°C. Line two baking sheets with parchment.

2. Use an electric stand mixer with a paddle attachment, beat the butter, canna-butter, brown sugar, and granulated sugar until smooth. Add the eggs and vanilla paste, and beat until incorporated and creamy.

3. In a separate bowl, combine the cake flour, all-purpose flour, baking powder, baking soda, and salt.

4. Add the dry ingredients to the wet ingredients and mix with quick spurts to incorporate. Add the chips and mix just enough to distribute them.

5. Divide the dough into 8 equal portions. Place 4 portions, flattened into discs on each prepared pan.

6. Bake the cookies for 11–13 minutes, or until they have turned golden. Don't overbake—that would be sad.

7. Let the cookies cool on the baking sheet for 5 minutes, then transfer to a wire rack and allow them to cool for at least 15 minutes more before enjoying.

Cannabis Coffee Cake Loaf

Yield: 1 loaf cake | Serving: 1 slice

THC: 5 milligrams per serving (45 milligrams total)

This cake is easy, and if you haven't done much baking, you will feel so good about yourself when you cut a slice and see the lovely streusel ripple running through the interior. It also tastes great and will definitely get you buzzed, if that's what you're going for.

CAKE

Baking spray

³/₄ cup sugar

7 tablespoons butter, room temperature

1½ tablespoons canna-butter, room temperature

2 large eggs, room temperature

2 teaspoons vanilla

½ cup sour cream

1¼ cups all-purpose flour

1 teaspoon baking powder

¼ teaspoon baking soda

¼ teaspoon salt

STREUSEL TOPPING

²/₃ cup flour

½ cup brown sugar

2 teaspoons cinnamon

²/₃ cup unsweetened, shredded coconut

½ cup mini chocolate chips

3 tablespoons unsalted butter, chilled and cubed

1. Heat the oven to 340°F/171°C. Spray a 9-by-5-inch loaf pan with baking spray.

2. Using an electric mixer, cream together the sugar, butter, and canna-butter until fluffy. Beat in the eggs, one at a time. Mix in the vanilla and sour cream until well combined.

3. In a separate bowl, combine the flour, baking powder, baking soda, and salt.

4. Add the dry ingredients to the wet ingredients and mix until just combined.

5. Make the streusel topping: In a medium bowl, combine all of the streusel ingredients. Mix with pastry cutter or clean hands until well combined and the butter is the size of small peas.

6. Pour half of the cake batter into the prepared loaf pan and top with half of the streusel mixture. Add the remaining batter and top with the remaining streusel mixture.

7. Bake for about 50–60 minutes or until a toothpick inserted into the center of the cake comes out clean. Cool and run a knife around the edges before removing it from the pan.

8. Allow to cool before cutting into nine 1-inch slices.

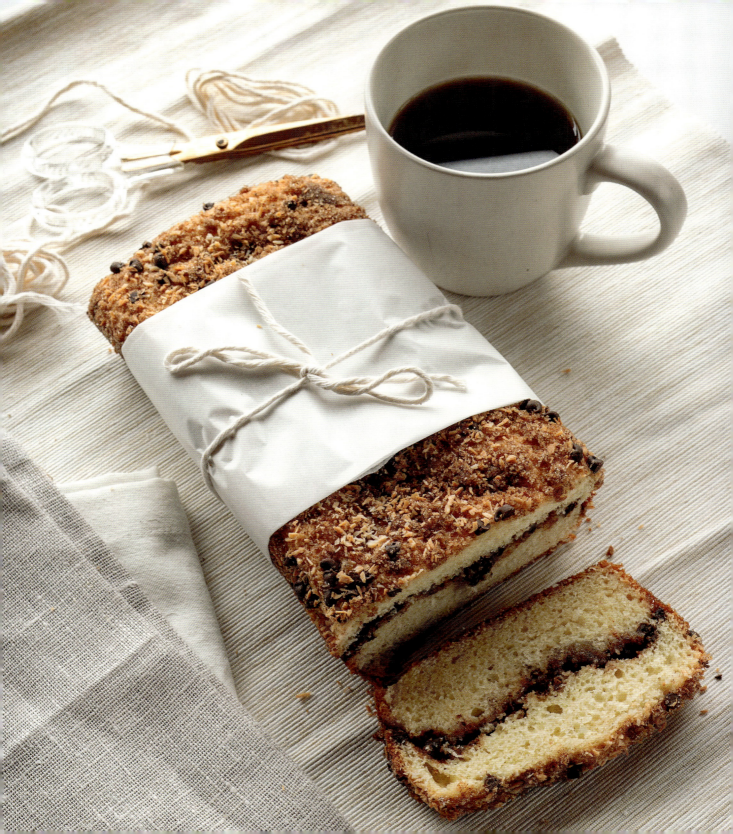

Nutter Lemon Cookies

Yield: 24 cookies | Serving: 1 cookie

THC: 5 milligrams per serving (120 milligrams total)

I'm not a lemon lover, but when it comes in a cookie with some white chocolate, it's a game changer. These cookies are lovely with a cup of tea, including a Thai tea (see page 134). Another lemon thing that I love is lemon curd, which is here, too (see page 176).

Baking spray

½ cup unsalted butter, room temperature

4 tablespoons canna-butter, room temperature

½ cup granulated sugar

½ cup light brown sugar, firmly packed

1 egg, room temperature

2 teaspoons vanilla extract

Zest from 1 lemon

1¾ cups all-purpose flour

½ teaspoon baking powder

Pinch salt

½ cup macadamia nuts, chopped

½ cup white chocolate chips, optional

1. Heat the oven to 325°F/163°C. Spray two baking sheets with cooking spray.

2. Using an electric mixer, combine the butter, canna-butter, sugar, brown sugar, egg, vanilla, and lemon zest and beat until light and creamy.

3. In a separate bowl, combine the flour, baking powder, and salt. Add the dry ingredients to the wet ingredients and mix until just combined. Add the nuts and chips and mix until distributed evenly.

4. Place the batter on the baking sheets in heaping tablespoons to form 24 cookies, at least 2 inches apart.

5. Bake the cookies until the edges are light golden brown, about 15–17 minutes. Allow to cool slightly before transferring to a cooling rack.

Chocolate Bark with Pretzels and Pecans

Yield: 12 pieces | Serving: 2 pieces

THC: 5 milligrams per serving (30 milligrams total)

Chocolate bark is often how I start a cannabis cooking class. Sometimes we open the kitchen and let people make their own. The Laurie + MaryJane kitchen becomes like a sundae bar for CBD bark. The choices of toppings are huge, and anything goes. This bark is so customizable and lots of fun to make. It also makes a great gift.

2 cups dark chocolate chips

2 tablespoons infused canna-butter

1 cup mini twist pretzels

½ cup pecan halves

½ unsweetened, shredded coconut

1. In a microwave-safe bowl, melt the chocolate chips. Start with 30 seconds and continue in 15-second intervals, stirring after each.

2. Add the canna-butter and stir to distribute evenly. Add the pretzels and pecans.

3. Place a piece of parchment on your work surface. Turn the chocolate mixture onto the parchment and spread using a spatula or spoon.

4. Allow to set for at least 45 minutes before breaking into 12 pieces.

5. Top each individual piece with a sprinkling of shredded coconut.

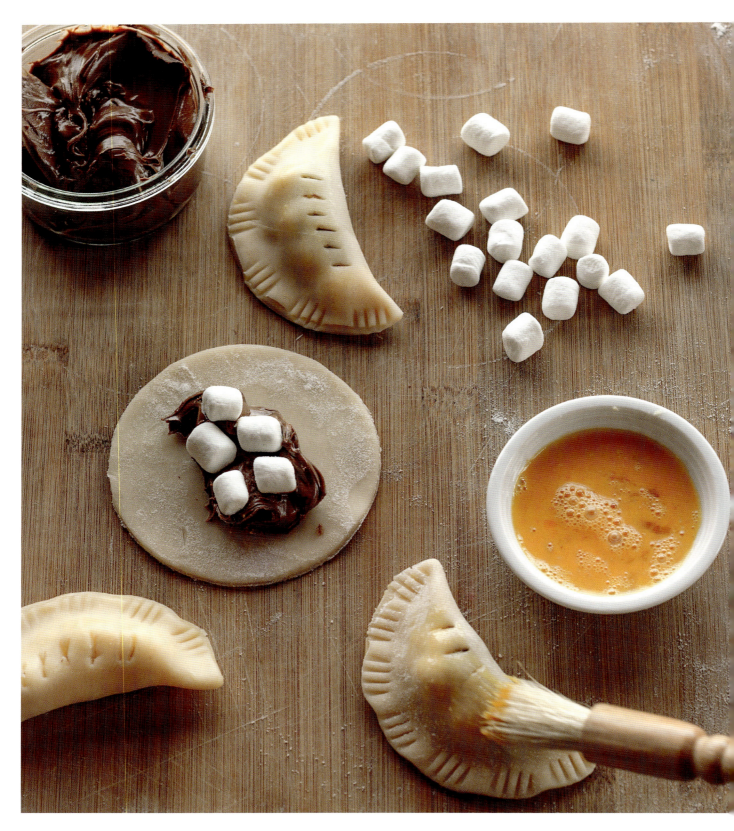

Nutella Marshmallow Hand Pies

Yield: 8 hand pies | Serving: 1 hand pie

THC: 5 milligrams per serving (40 milligrams total)

There's no denying that this is a decadent pie, but man, it is so, so good. I will admit to taking a jar of that hazelnut spread, plopping myself in front of the telly, and eating the whole thing. And I'm not talking about the small jar. If you're not in the mood for an entire pie, just infuse the hazelnut spread and stir it into some coffee.

2 refrigerated piecrusts

Flour, for dusting

4 teaspoons canna-butter, melted

1 cup chocolate-hazelnut spread

1 cup marshmallow spread, or 40 mini marshmallows

1 egg, lightly beaten

1. Heat the oven to 340°F/171°C. Line two baking sheets with parchment paper.

2. Place the piecrusts on a floured work surface and roll them out slightly to a bit more than 12 inches in diameter. Cut out eight 4-inch circles (use a bowl for a template).

3. Mix the melted canna-butter with the chocolate-hazelnut spread.

4. Evenly distribute the chocolate-hazelnut spread among the circles and spread, leaving a $^{1}/_{2}$-inch rim around the edge of each circle. Repeat with the marshmallow spread.

5. Using a pastry brush, paint the edges of the circles with the beaten egg. Fold the crust over and press to seal. Using a fork, make indentations around the edge of the crust. With a sharp knife, cut a few vents for steam in the body of each pie.

6. Bake the hand pies for 12–14 minutes or until golden brown. Allow to cool briefly before eating.

Cherry Crostata

Yield: 9 slices | Serving: 1 slice

THC: 5 milligrams per serving (45 milligrams total)

This flaky crust pairs beautifully with the sweet and tart cherry filling. A crostata is a freeform pie, which means it's very forgiving and also fun to make. You can pick the fruit based on whatever is in season, or go with frozen. Besides cherry, my other favorite versions of this crostata use peach and blueberry.

1^3/$_4$ cups all-purpose flour, plus more for the work surface

5 tablespoons sugar, divided

^{1}/$_2$ teaspoon cinnamon

Pinch salt

12 tablespoons cold unsalted butter, divided

1^1/$_2$ tablespoons cold canna-butter

5 tablespoons ice water

1 pound cherries, pitted (frozen works, too)

1 tablespoon cornstarch

2 tablespoons orange juice

2 teaspoons lemon juice

Zest of 1 orange

Coarse sugar, for dusting

1. In a food processor, combine the flour, 3 tablespoons of the sugar, cinnamon, and salt. Cut up 8 tablespoons of the butter into pieces. Add it to the food processor along with the canna-butter and pulse until pea-size crumbs form.

2. Add the ice water and pulse until the dough comes together. Wrap in plastic wrap and chill for 1 hour.

3. In a separate bowl, combine the cherries, the remaining 2 tablespoons of sugar, cornstarch, orange juice, lemon juice, and orange zest.

4. Heat the oven to 340°F/171°C. On a lightly floured surface, roll the dough into a circle ^{1}/$_8$ inch thick. Place the fruit on the crust, leaving a 1^1/$_2$ inch border. Fold the crust up around the edges of the fruit. Cut the remaining 4 tablespoons of butter into small pieces and distribute them over the fruit. Sprinkle coarse sugar over the crostata.

5. Bake for 35–40 minutes, until the crust has browned and the fruit is bubbling.

6. Once cooled, slice into 9 pieces and serve.

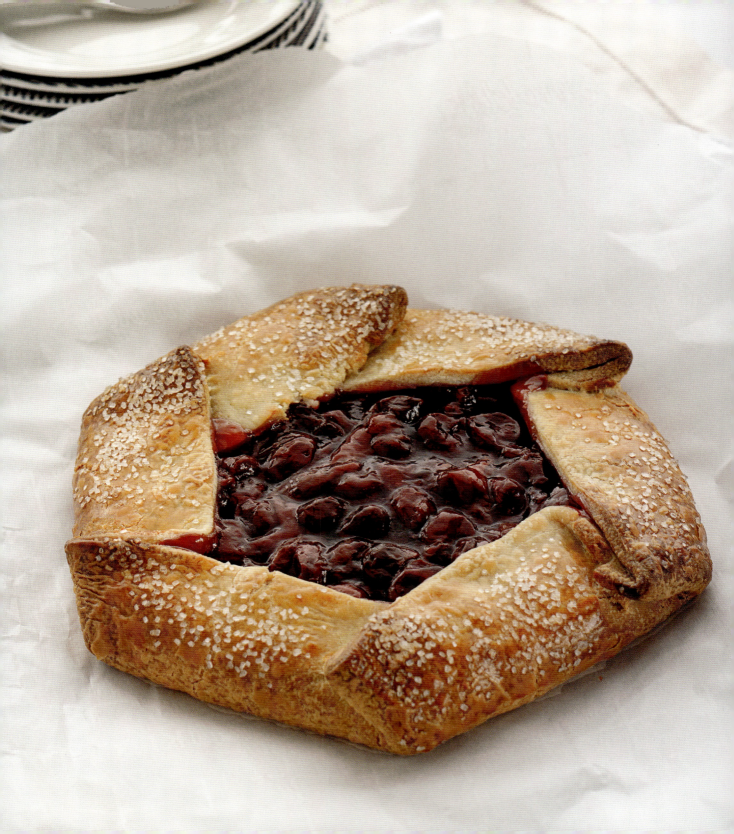

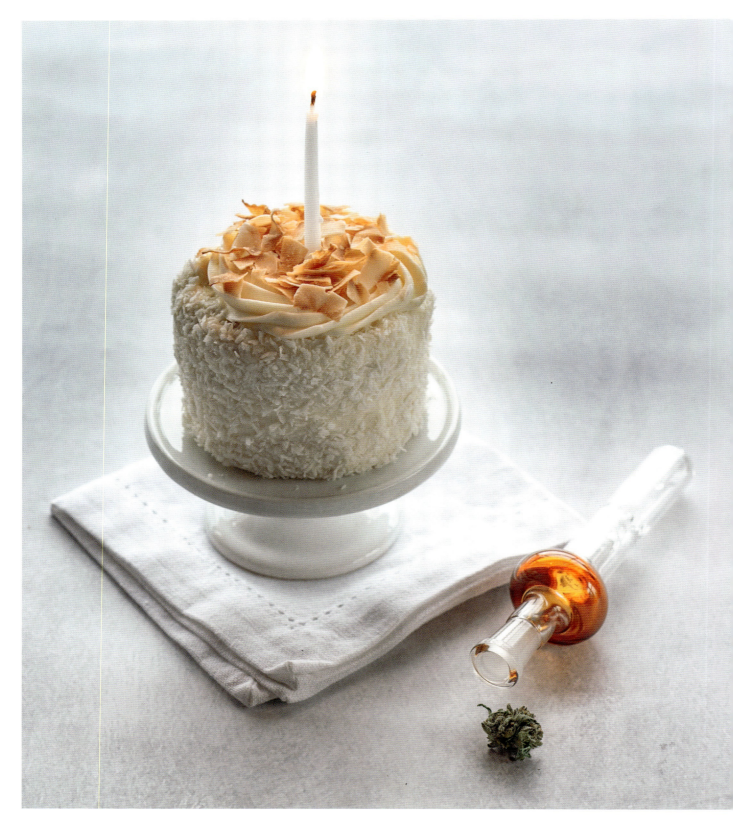

Birthday Cake

Yield: One 4-inch double-layer cake (8 slices) | Serving: 1 slice
THC: 5 milligrams per serving (20 milligrams total)

This mini cake is just right for a small gathering or for a solo celebration with leftovers. Infused with CBD oil, this cake will make sure you enjoy your special day. Should you go the THC route, it might be best to stay home and stare at the balloons.

CAKE
Baking spray

½ cup cake flour

⅔ cup sugar

½ teaspoon baking soda

¼ teaspoon baking powder

⅛ teaspoon salt

⅓ cup sour cream

⅓ cup cold coffee

1 egg, room temperature

2 tablespoons vegetable oil

4 teaspoons infused oil or butter, melted

1 teaspoon vanilla extract

FROSTING
½ cup butter, softened

2 cups powdered sugar, sifted

2 teaspoons vanilla

2 tablespoons heavy cream

1–2 cups unsweetened, shredded coconut

¼ cup toasted coconut flakes

1. Heat the oven to 340°F/171°C. Spray two 4-inch cake pans with nonstick baking spray.

2. For the cake: In a large bowl, combine the flour, sugar, baking soda, baking powder, and salt. Using a mixer, beat the sour cream, coffee, egg, vegetable oil, the infused oil, and vanilla until well mixed. Add the dry ingredients and mix until just combined.

3. Divide the batter between the two pans. Bake until a toothpick inserted in the center comes out clean, about 25–30 minutes. Allow to cool on a rack.

4. For the frosting: In a mixing bowl, combine the butter, sugar, vanilla, and cream. Beat until fluffy, 5–7 minutes.

5. Place one layer of the cooled cake on a plate. Spread frosting on top of the layer. Place the second layer on top of the first. Spread the remaining frosting around the top and sides of the cake, leaving 2 tablespoons of frosting in a mound on the top center for decoration.

6. Press the unsweetened coconut into the frosting, trying to get it all over as evenly as possible. Sprinkle the top of the cake with the toasted coconut flakes. Chill for at least 1 hour before serving. Happy birthday!

Savory Recipes

Rosemary Chips with Infused Onion Dip

Yield: About 4 cups dip, with homemade chips | Servings: 12 (¹/₃ cup dip per serving)

THC: 5 milligrams per serving

———————————

There's not a whole lot more satisfying in the world than crispy chips, or fries, or chips but "not those kind," as they say in other places. Regardless of what place you might be in, you have the option to make these thicker or thinner to oblige the craving.

ROSEMARY CHIPS

Baking spray

3 russet potatoes

3 tablespoons extra virgin olive oil

1½ tablespoons fresh rosemary, chopped

1½ teaspoons salt

1 teaspoon coarse black pepper

INFUSED ONION DIP

2 tablespoons unsalted butter

2 tablespoons canna-butter

¼ cup canola oil

2 large yellow onions, peeled and sliced ⅛-inch thick

½ teaspoon salt

½ teaspoon black pepper

Pinch of cayenne

4 ounces cream cheese, softened

1 cup sour cream, room temperature

ROSEMARY CHIPS

1. Heat oven to 425°F/218°C. Spray two cookie sheets with sides, or line with parchment.

2. Place the potatoes on your work surface. Thinly slice or cut in wedges. Place in a large Ziploc bag.

3. Add the remaining ingredients to the bag and manipulate the bag so that the potatoes are evenly coated.

4. Bake the chips until crisp, about 10–12 minutes, turning once halfway through the cooking process.

INFUSED ONION DIP

1. In a large saucepan, heat the butters and oil. Add the onions and spices and sauté, slowly, until the onions are well caramelized. Allow to cool.

2. In the bowl of a food processor, combine the onions with the cream cheese and sour cream. Process till smooth. Taste for salt and pepper, and chill for a minimum of 1 hour.

Naan with Goat Cheese and Arugula

Yield: 2 pieces | Servings: 2 (1 piece per serving)
THC: 5 milligrams per serving

The first time I had freshly made ricotta was in Italy while I was working on a cookbook with renowned chef Giuliano Bugialli. We were in a tiny town and had dinner in a terrific restaurant. My pasta had a red sauce topped with a lemony fresh ricotta. Wow, that was a moment. This combination of flavors and textures is complex and exquisite.

1 piece large naan (approximately 4 ounces) lightly toasted, cut in half

8 tablespoons goat cheese, room temperature

1 teaspoon canna-oil or melted canna-butter

2 teaspoons freshly grated lemon zest

1 small bunch baby arugula, rinsed and patted dry

3 tablespoons vinaigrette of choice

2 tablespoons chopped fresh parsley

1 teaspoon Aleppo pepper

½ teaspoon coarse salt

1–2 tablespoons honey

2 tablespoons, plus 1 teaspoon good-quality olive oil

Lemon wedges, optional

1. Place the naan on your work surface.

2. Mix canna-oil or canna-butter with the goat cheese. Spread evenly on each piece of naan.

3. In a medium bowl, combine the lemon zest, arugula, vinaigrette, parsley, pepper, and salt.

4. Divide the mixture between the 2 pieces of bread.

5. Just before serving, drizzle each piece with the honey and olive oil. Serve with lemon wedges for an optional topping.

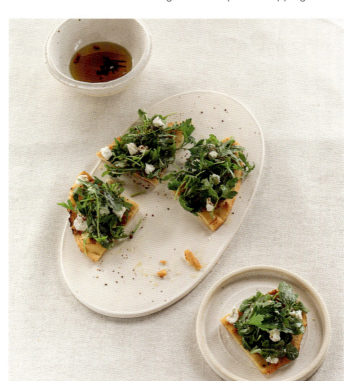

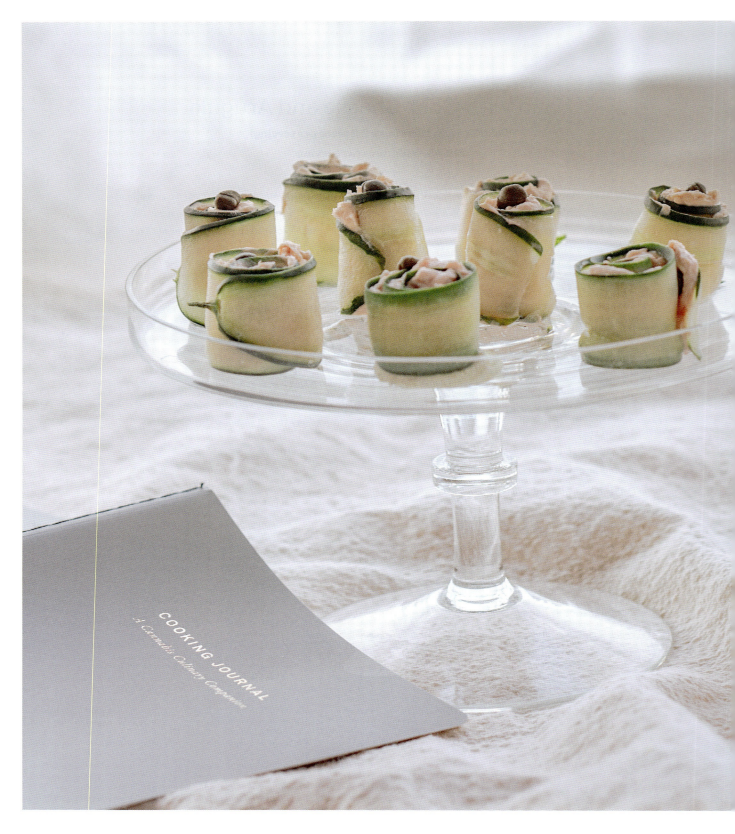

Cucumber Spirals

Yield: 16 pieces | Servings: 8 (2 pieces per serving)
THC: 5 milligrams per serving (2.5 milligrams per piece)

If you're at all like me, even a little bit, you see those premade wrap platters at the grocery store and think, "I can make that so much better" . . . then you buy it anyway? This recipe is for the self-motivator that wants to put the premade platter producer to shame. Not only are the flavors in this dish so amazing together, they also perk your taste buds right up.

2 cucumbers, ends cut off

4 teaspoons canna-butter

8 ounces cream cheese, softened

4 ounces smoked salmon

4 tablespoons mayonnaise

1 scallion, cut in ¼-inch pieces

2 tablespoons chopped dill

1 tablespoon fresh lemon juice

½ teaspoon black pepper

½ teaspoon salt

3 tablespoons capers

1. Place the cucumbers on your work surface. Using a vegetable peeler, slice the cucumbers the long way, trying to cut a slice that is the full length of the cucumber. Pat the slices dry with a clean dish towel or paper towels.

2. In a food processor, combine the canna-butter, cream cheese, salmon, mayonnaise, scallion, dill, lemon juice, pepper, and salt. Pulse until a semismooth consistency is reached.

3. Slather each slice with the spread, 1–2 tablespoons each. Sprinkle with the capers. Tightly roll each slice. The slices will stay together due to the spread. Place on a serving tray and enjoy.

Poppers and Gouda

Yield: 12 poppers | Servings: 6 (2 poppers per serving)
THC: 5 milligrams per serving (2.5 milligrams per popper)

Jalapeño poppers are the best comfort food when you want revenge on your spicy-intolerant family member. Just kidding! This recipe is so perfect for bringing yourself back to life—the spiciness can be your friend or your enemy, so take out more seeds for the mildest experience or leave in more seeds if you just feel dead inside.

6 jalapeño peppers, cut in half and seeded

2 ounces cream cheese, softened

1 cup shredded gouda

1 tablespoon canna-butter, melted and cooled

½ teaspoon smoked paprika

¼ teaspoon ground cumin

½ teaspoon salt

3 scallions

1. Heat oven to 340°F/171°C. Line a baking sheet with parchment paper.

2. Cut the peppers in half, and remove the seeds with a spoon. Don't touch your eyes without washing your hands first—the jalapeños sting!

3. In a small bowl, stir together the cream cheese, gouda, butter, paprika, cumin, and salt until well mixed.

4. Divide the filling evenly between the pepper halves. Cut the scallions in half the long way, removing the white ends while keeping the green ends. Wrap a scallion around each pepper half, and secure with a toothpick if needed.

5. Bake until the cheese is melted, and the scallion is soft and lightly browned, about 15 minutes.

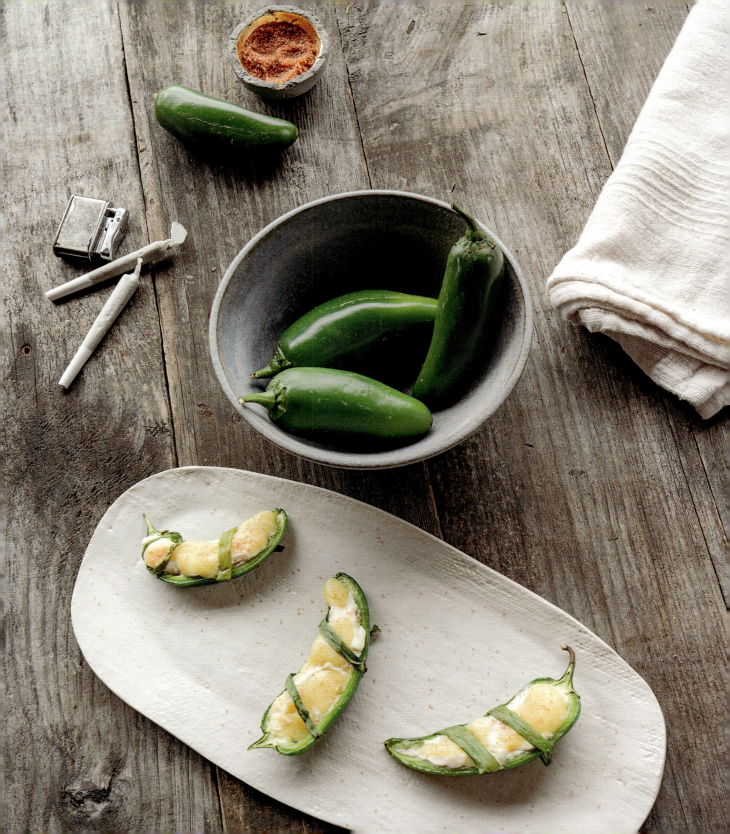

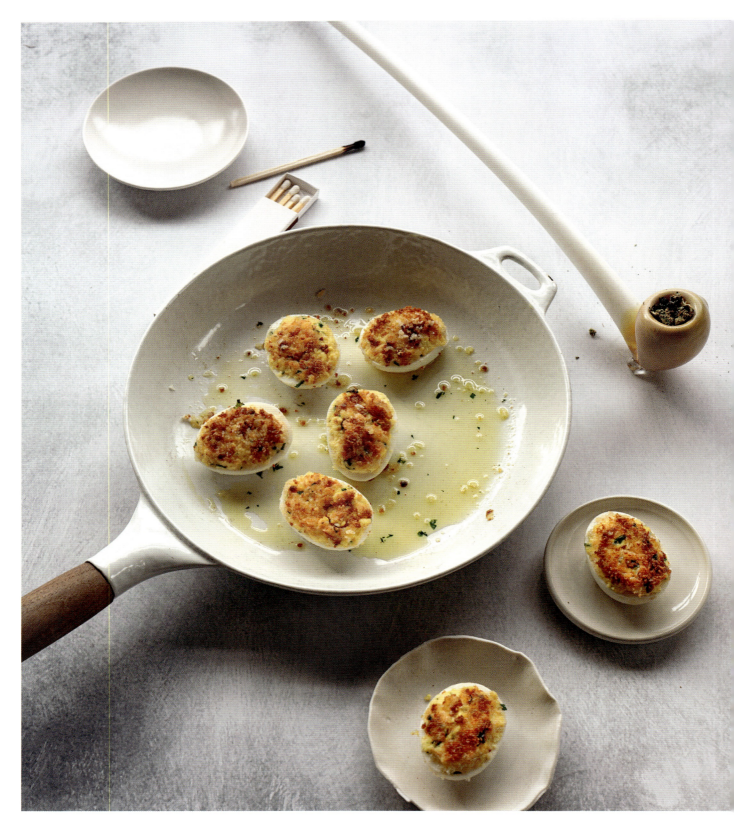

Panko Griddled Deviled Eggs

Yield: 12 deviled eggs | Servings: 6 (2 deviled eggs per serving)
THC: 5 milligrams per serving (2.5 milligrams per deviled egg)

Truly one of my favorite recipes, this griddled deviled egg is off-the-charts fantastic. When eating a deviled egg with a buttery panko crust, I have to use considerable restraint, and I think you will, too. I have made these eggs with brioche crumbs as well, and I would do it again.

6 hard-boiled eggs, peeled and cut in half

2 tablespoons mayonnaise

1 tablespoon sour cream

1 tablespoon canna-butter, melted and cooled

1 tablespoon finely chopped scallion

1 tablespoon finely chopped parsley

2 teaspoons Dijon mustard

1 teaspoon horseradish

½ teaspoon lemon juice

½ teaspoon salt

¼ teaspoon coarse black pepper

1–2 cups panko bread crumbs

2 tablespoons unsalted butter

1. Place the egg halves on your work surface. Remove the yolks, and place them in a medium bowl.

2. Add the mayonnaise, sour cream, butter, scallion, parsley, mustard, horseradish, lemon juice, salt, and pepper to the bowl. Mash all the ingredients and combine until smooth.

3. Divide the mixture between the egg halves. If you like a smoother consistency, then piping the mixture with a piping bag is a great idea. For a chunkier version, feel free to scoop and fill the egg halves with a spoon. Chill for 30 minutes.

4. Remove the eggs from the fridge. Place bread crumbs into a shallow dish. One by one, dip the egg (filling side down) in the bread crumbs.

5. Heat a nonstick skillet over medium heat with butter.

6. Place the eggs in a pan, crumbs side down, and sauté until golden brown, 5-7 minutes. Carefully turn the eggs to let them heat for 1-2 minutes on the underside. Carefully remove with a spatula. Serve warm.

Mushroom Fontina Tart

Yield: 9 slices | Servings: 9 (1 slice per serving) | THC: 5 milligrams per serving

Melted Fontina cheese is dreamy. Very creamy, gentle, and buttery, it raises the bar considerably on a grilled cheese sandwich, and this easy-to-put-together savory tart will become a favorite. I have made the tart with both roasted peppers and asparagus with excellent results.

1 sheet frozen puff pastry, defrosted according to package directions

1½ tablespoons canna-butter

2 tablespoons unsalted butter

1 leek, peeled and thinly sliced

1 clove garlic, finely chopped

1 teaspoon fresh thyme

2 cups mushrooms, trimmed and sliced

6 slices bacon, cooked lightly and chopped

1½ cups grated or chopped Fontina cheese

Salt and pepper, to taste

¼ cup chopped scallions

1. Heat oven to 340°F/171°C.

2. Place the puff pastry on a floured work surface, and roll out an additional 1–2 inches. Place on a parchment–lined baking sheet, and chill.

3. In a large sauté pan, heat the butters over medium heat. When temperature is relatively hot, add the leek, garlic, and thyme, and sauté until tender, 5–6 minutes. Remove from heat, and place ingredients on a plate.

4. Add the mushrooms, and cook until done, 7–9 minutes; their liquid will release, simmer away, and turn golden with sautéing.

5. Spread the leek, mushrooms, and bacon over the pastry. Sprinkle with the cheese, and follow with the salt and pepper.

6. Bake until the cheese is melted and the tart is golden brown, about 25–30 minutes. Sprinkle with remaining scallions.

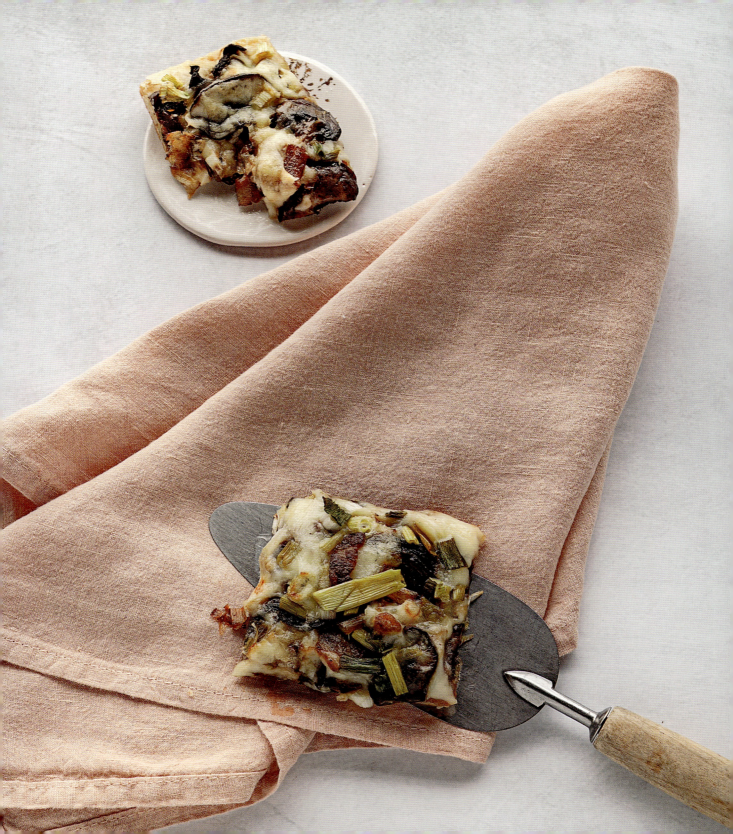

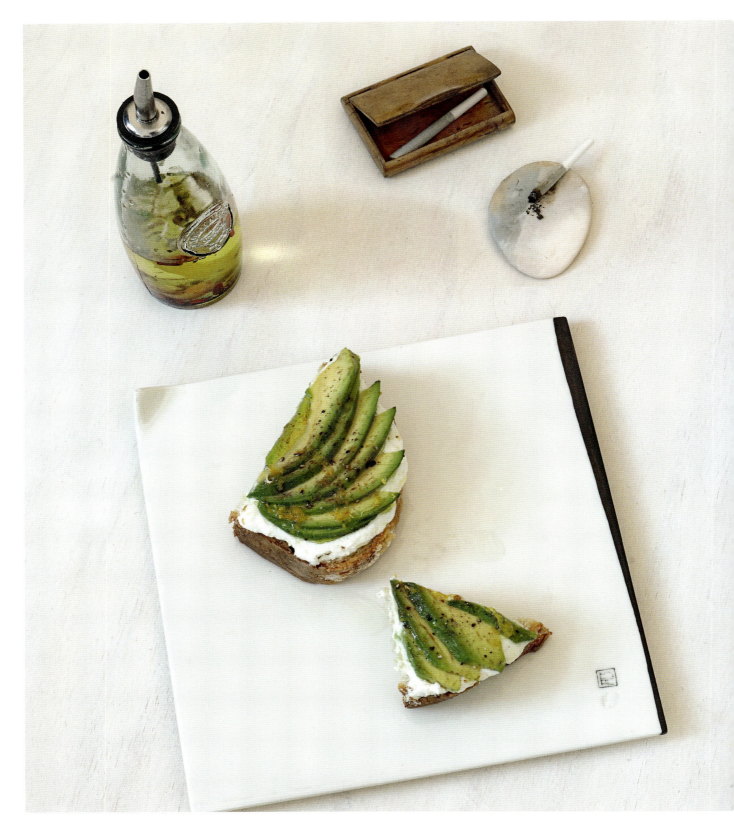

Citrus Avocado Ricotta Bruschetta

Yield: 2 pieces of bruschetta | Servings: 2 (1 piece per serving)

THC: 10 milligrams per serving

When all else fails, eat carbs and fruit. The name's a mouthful, so it's pretty fun when you say it three times fast—Citrus Avocado Ricotta Bruschetta, Citrus Avocado Ricotta Bruschetta, Citrus Avocado Ric . . . you get it.

I find happiness in this recipe because it hits all the flavors you want in such a nice way. Tartness and sweetness from the orange juice, richness from the avocado, a kick from the pepper. You really can't hide from the happiness this recipe brings you—you know, unless you're actively avoiding happiness.

2 (½-inch thick) crusty country bread slices, toasted

1 teaspoon canna-oil

½ cup ricotta (see the following recipe)

2 teaspoons orange juice with pulp

¼ teaspoon salt

¼ teaspoon coarse black pepper

1 teaspoon orange zest

1 tablespoon olive oil, plus oil for drizzle

1 avocado, peeled and pitted and thinly sliced

1. Place the bread on your work surface. Brush the bread with the oil. Divide the ricotta over the 2 bread slices.

2. In a small bowl, whisk together the orange juice, salt, pepper, zest, and 1 tablespoon olive oil.

3. Toss the avocado slices with the orange mixture. Place the avocado slices on top of the ricotta. Drizzle with additional oil if desired.

RICOTTA

My friend Megan, a terrific chef, gave me this ricotta recipe. Now I try to always have fresh ricotta in the fridge, considering there are so many ways to enjoy it. It's quite a bit better than the kind you can buy in the supermarket, though in this dish, with the powerful flavor palate, you will be fine going with store-bought. I have it with fresh fruit and cannabis or I dollop it on pasta with cannabis, and it never disappoints.

RICOTTA

1 cup heavy cream

3 cups whole milk

1½ cups buttermilk

1. Mix all the ingredients in a pot and stir. Bring to a simmer, and allow the curds to form. Do not let it come to a full boil. You will see the curds floating up to the surface. All it takes is 10–15 minutes! Strain through a chinois or cheesecloth, and chill well.

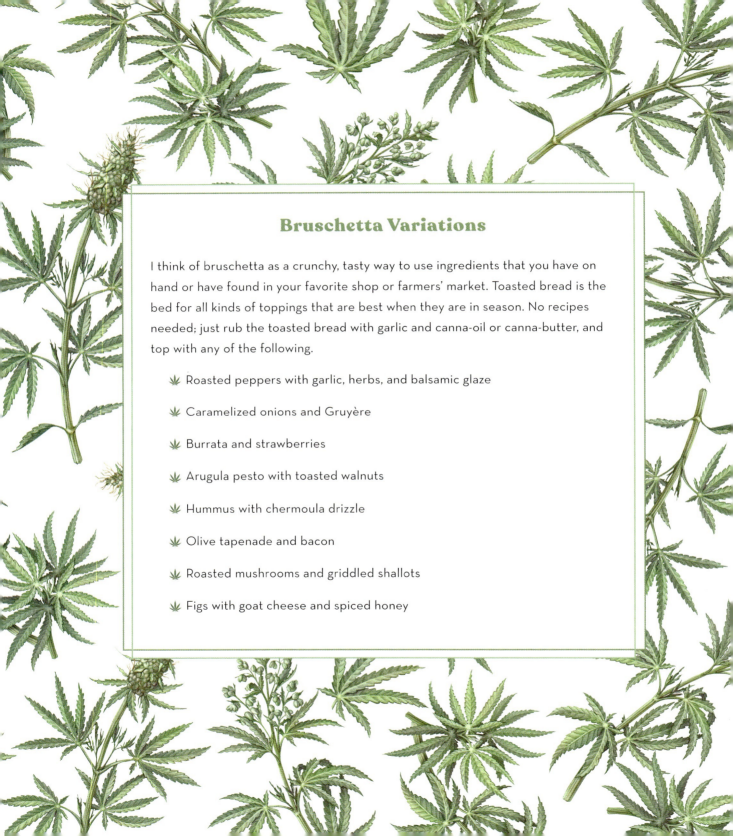

Bruschetta Variations

I think of bruschetta as a crunchy, tasty way to use ingredients that you have on hand or have found in your favorite shop or farmers' market. Toasted bread is the bed for all kinds of toppings that are best when they are in season. No recipes needed; just rub the toasted bread with garlic and canna-oil or canna-butter, and top with any of the following.

- Roasted peppers with garlic, herbs, and balsamic glaze

- Caramelized onions and Gruyère

- Burrata and strawberries

- Arugula pesto with toasted walnuts

- Hummus with chermoula drizzle

- Olive tapenade and bacon

- Roasted mushrooms and griddled shallots

- Figs with goat cheese and spiced honey

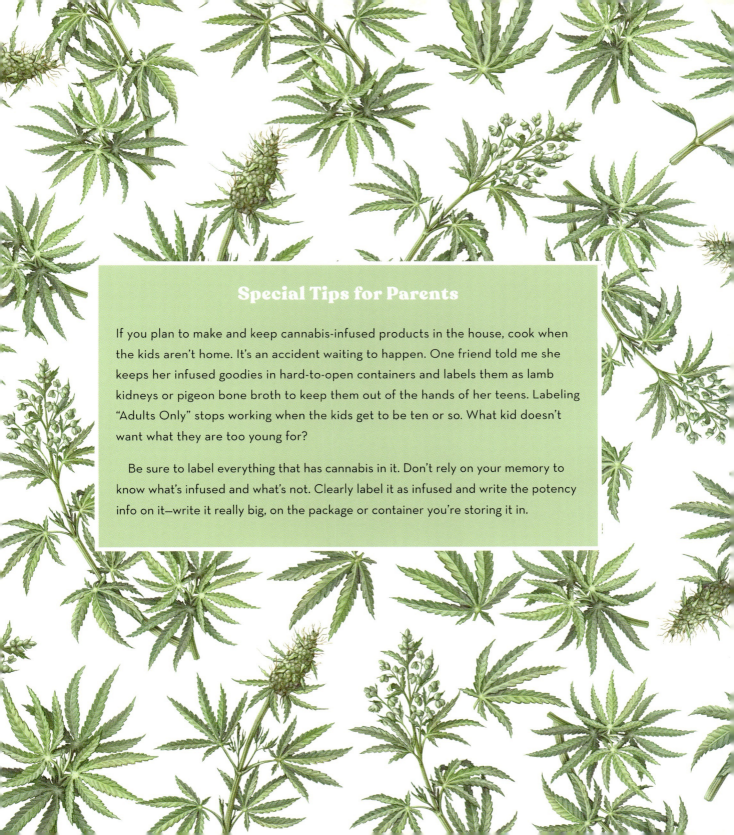

Special Tips for Parents

If you plan to make and keep cannabis-infused products in the house, cook when the kids aren't home. It's an accident waiting to happen. One friend told me she keeps her infused goodies in hard-to-open containers and labels them as lamb kidneys or pigeon bone broth to keep them out of the hands of her teens. Labeling "Adults Only" stops working when the kids get to be ten or so. What kid doesn't want what they are too young for?

Be sure to label everything that has cannabis in it. Don't rely on your memory to know what's infused and what's not. Clearly label it as infused and write the potency info on it—write it really big, on the package or container you're storing it in.

Hummus Cucumber Sandwich

Yield: 1 sandwich | Serving: 1 sandwich | THC: 5 milligrams per serving

A cannabis book without a hummus recipe seems wrong. This time we're putting it on a sandwich with some other good stuff. There's a lot going on in this sandwich, and each element adds a special something.

8-inch piece of baguette, sliced in half

⅓ cup hummus

1 teaspoon canna-oil

½ cup salad greens

6 thin cucumber slices

2 pieces roasted red pepper

4–6 spinach leaves

1. Place the baguette slices on a work surface. In a small bowl, mix the hummus with the canna-oil. Spread a slice of bread with the hummus.

2. Top the hummus with the greens, cucumber slices, red pepper, and spinach.

3. Top with the remaining slice of bread. Cut the sandwich on the diagonal.

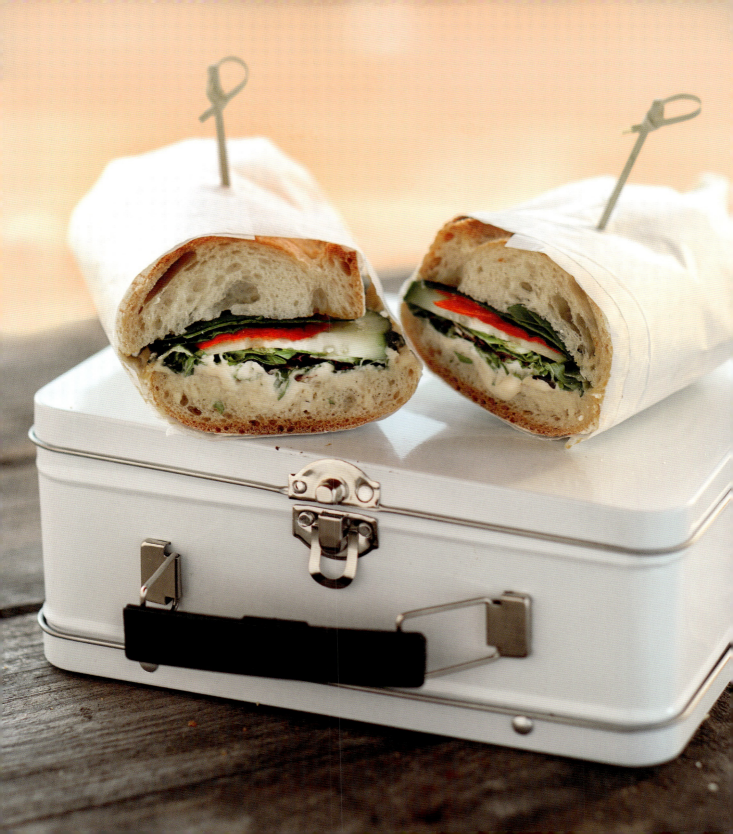

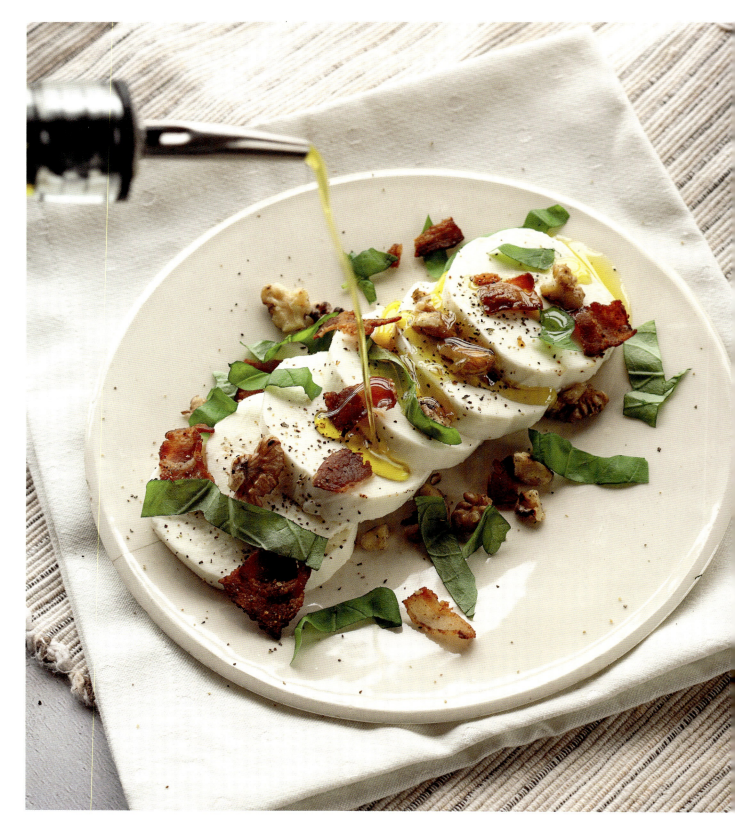

Fresh Mozzarella with Cannabis Drizzle

Yield: 9 slices | Serving: 3 slices

THC: 5 milligrams per serving (15 milligrams total)

This use of mozzarella does not require a perfectly ripe tomato, so it's great in any season. I make this as a starter year round, and everyone loves it. If mozzarella only speaks to you when combined with tomato, then during the cold months I suggest roasting cherry tomatoes in olive oil and add them to this recipe. Either way, this recipe is quite tasty.

9 slices good-quality fresh mozzarella cheese

6 basil leaves, shredded

2 strips bacon, cooked until crisp and chopped

2 tablespoons toasted chopped walnuts

2 tablespoons olive oil

1½ teaspoon canna-olive oil

1 clove garlic, minced

Coarse black pepper

Crusty bread, for serving

1. Arrange the mozzarella slices on a small plate. Sprinkle with the basil, bacon, and walnuts.

2. Combine the olive oil and canna-olive oil with the garlic and drizzle over the mozzarella. Season with pepper.

3. Serve with crusty bread.

Garbanzos for the Road

Yield: 5 cups | Serving: 1 ¼ cups

THC: 5 milligrams per serving (20 milligrams total)

———

Sometimes I make this salad with CBD and then bring it to work for lunch. Somehow, I always end up sharing. If I make this version with a THC infusion, folks have to come to my house to eat it, and they have to promise to stay until the effects of the THC are gone. This salad is healthy and good for you, and it only gets better as the flavors comingle. If you're looking for a more substantial meal, add chicken, tofu, or shrimp.

2 tablespoons cider vinegar

2 tablespoons olive oil

2 teaspoons canna-olive oil

1 tablespoon lime juice

2 teaspoons curry powder

1 teaspoon salt

1 teaspoon cumin

½ teaspoon turmeric

½ teaspoon Aleppo pepper

3 (15.5-ounce) cans chickpeas (aka garbanzo beans), rinsed and drained

2 grilled chicken breasts, thinly sliced

1 cup shredded carrots

Pita chips

1. In a large bowl, combine the vinegar, olive oil, canna-olive oil, lime juice, curry powder, salt, cumin, turmeric, Aleppo pepper, chickpeas, chicken, and carrots and mix well to combine flavors. Allow to sit for 30 minutes before serving.

2. Serve with pita chips. I like to mix them into the salad. Dressing and crunch—perfect together.

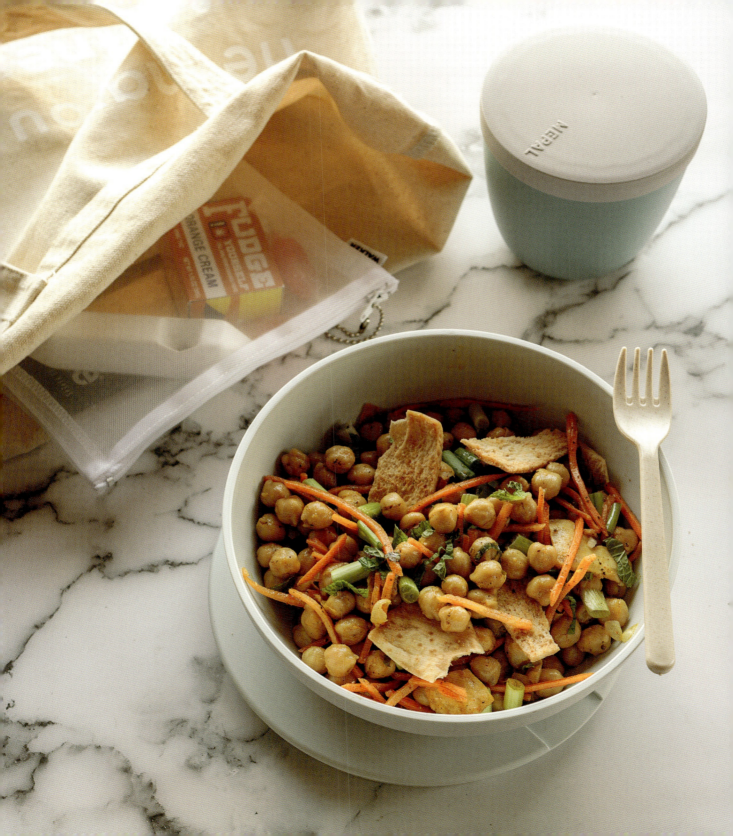

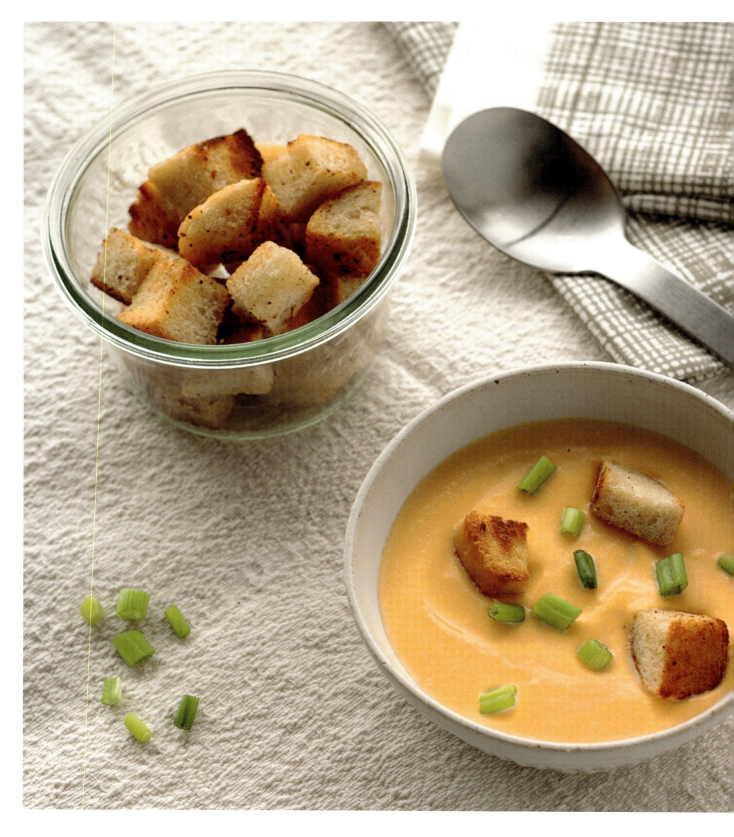

Spicy Sweet Potato Soup

Yield: 6 cups | Serving: 1 cup

THC: 5 milligrams per serving (30 milligrams total)

This soup helped me to fall in love with sweet potatoes and yams. The roasting adds caramelization, and the smoked paprika gives this a complexity that you will love. I don't think I'll ever want sweet potatoes covered with marshmallows, but this is my rainy day soup. Because I live in Oregon, that means I eat a lot of this soup!

4 large sweet potatoes

2 tablespoons extra virgin olive oil

1 large onion, peeled and sliced

1 large carrot, peeled and sliced

2 garlic cloves, minced

1 teaspoon smoked paprika

½ teaspoon cumin

½ teaspoon salt

1 cup half-and-half

1 tablespoon canna-butter

2 tablespoons scallions, sliced

Croutons,* for serving

1. Heat the oven to 400°F/204°C.

2. Pierce each sweet potato several times with a fork. Place them on a baking sheet and roast until tender, 45–60 minutes.

3. Meanwhile, in a large skillet over medium heat, heat the olive oil. Add the onion, carrot, garlic, paprika, cumin, and salt and cook until the carrots are tender, about 15 minutes. Add the mixture to a food processor or blender along with the half-and-half and puree until smooth. Place the mixture in a large saucepan and set it aside.

4. When the potatoes are done and slightly cooled, peel and dice them. Place the potatoes and canna-butter in the food processor and process until smooth.

5. Add the potato mixture to the saucepan and stir to combine. Place the saucepan over low heat and warm the soup, stirring frequently.

6. Serve topped with the scallions and croutons.

> * You have a choice here. If you want to infuse the croutons for a double dose, sauté the cubed bread in canna-butter until golden brown. If you want them unadulterated, just sauté the croutons in regular butter or oil. I always keep a jar of infused croutons in the house for last-minute additions.

Lemon Garlic Chicken Skewers

Yield: 8 skewers | Serving: 2 skewers | THC: 5 milligrams per serving

These skewers are full of flavor. The citrus, garlic, and coarse black pepper create a fresh, bright flavor palate. Sometimes, I like to take the food off the skewers and wrap it in lettuce leaves.

CHICKEN

2 large boneless, skinless chicken breasts, cut into 1-inch chunks

1 tablespoon fresh lemon juice

2 garlic cloves, minced

1 teaspoon coarse ground black pepper

¼ teaspoon salt

1 zucchini, sliced

8–12 whole mini sweet peppers

8 metal or wooden* skewers

SAUCE

2 teaspoons infused olive oil

½ cup plain Greek yogurt

1 tablespoon finely chopped bell pepper

1 teaspoon lemon juice

1 teaspoon turmeric

½ teaspoon ground cumin

¼ teaspoon ground ginger

1 garlic clove, minced

Pinch salt

1. Preheat the grill.

2. In a medium bowl, mix the chicken pieces with 1 tablespoon of the lemon juice, minced garlic, pepper, and salt. Allow the chicken to marinate for 30 minutes.

3. Thread the chicken pieces, zucchini slices, and mini peppers on the skewers, alternating to your liking.

4. In a small bowl, combine the infused olive oil, yogurt, chopped bell pepper, the remaining teaspoon of lemon juice, turmeric, ginger, additional minced garlic, and a pinch of salt. Stir well.

5. Grill the skewers until the chicken is no longer pink and its juices run clear.

6. Serve chicken skewers with the sauce on the side for dipping, and with lettuce if so desired.

> * If you are using wooden skewers, be sure to soak them in water for at least 30 minutes before putting them on the grill. Also, be sure to let the grill heat up before cooking, as this will decrease the chance of the food sticking.

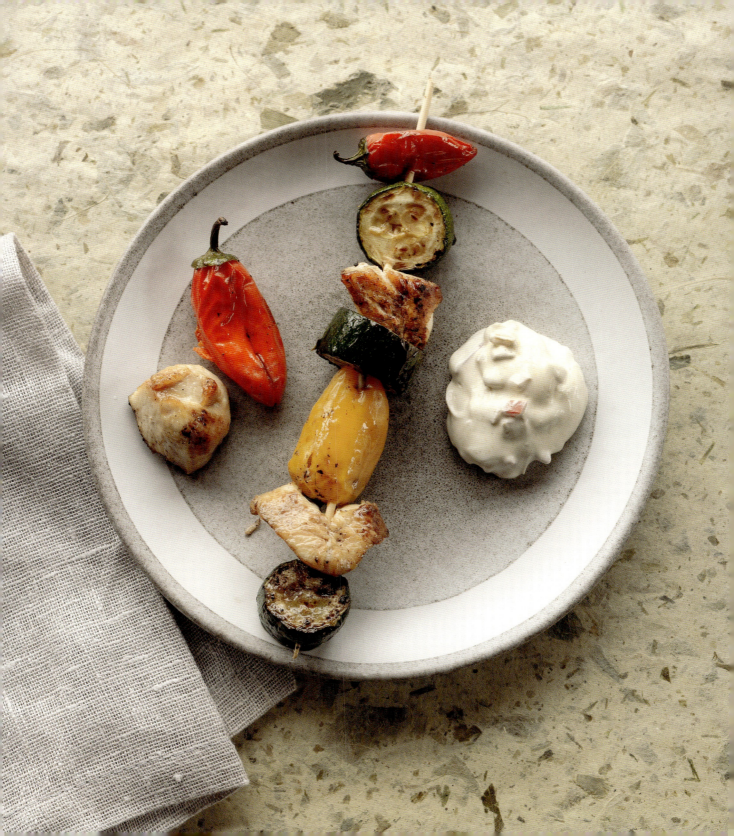

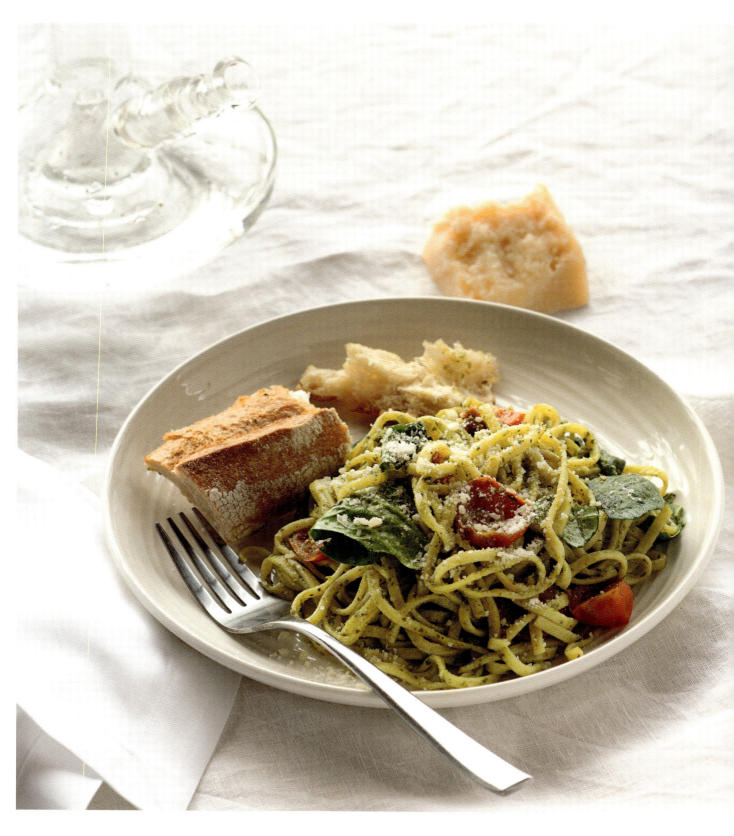

Linguine Spinach and Pesto

Yield: 8 cups | Serving: 2 cups per person

THC: 5 milligrams per serving (20 milligrams total)

During the summer, I make and freeze several types of pesto: spinach, arugula, even kale! Pesto is so easy to infuse and it really does mask the taste of cannabis. What small cannabis taste does come through in this dish mixes very well with the other flavors. I tend to use a lot more garlic than I've called for below, but I think I use too much. Stick with the four cloves. Also, if I'm having trouble finding good cherry tomatoes, I roast them in a hot oven with a little olive oil for about eight minutes to help enhance their flavor.

PESTO

6 cups spinach, cleaned, dried, and packed

½ cup whole roasted almonds

4 cloves garlic, peeled

Salt

Pepper

½ cup olive oil

2 teaspoons infused olive oil

¼ cup grated Romano cheese

PASTA

1 pound pasta

1 bunch spinach, rinsed and dried on a clean dish towel

12 cherry tomatoes, halved

2 tablespoons olive oil

Small chunk Parmesan, for grating

1. In a food processor or blender, combine the spinach, almonds, garlic, salt, and pepper.

2. Drizzle in the olive oil and the infused olive oil.

3. Scrape the pesto into a bowl and stir in the cheese.

4. In a large pot, bring salted water to a boil. Cook the pasta according to the package instructions.

5. Drain the pasta, return it to the pot off the heat, and toss with the tomatoes, pesto, and spinach.

6. Divide the pasta among 4 plates, drizzle with olive oil, and grate some Parmesan over top.

Damn Good Dog Biscuits (CBD Biscuits)

Yield: 40 biscuits | Serving: 2 biscuits

CBD: 5 milligrams per serving (100 milligrams total)

Why not let Fido have a little fun? CBD for dogs is a growing trend. If you have a very active puppy who could use a little mellowing, or an older dog with sore joints, CBD can really be a lifesaver. This treat offers a good starting dose for most dogs, regardless of their size. If your dog requires a stronger dose, keep the recipe the same but add more CBD oil. When determining how large a dose of CBD to give your dog, I always suggest following the same procedure that I use for people: Start with a low dose and work your way up.

1 cup pumpkin or sweet potato puree

½ cup peanut butter

2 large eggs

2½ cups oats

¼ cup grated or shredded carrot

3 tablespoons plus 1 teaspoon CBD-infused coconut oil

¼ cup water

Chopped bacon, optional

Grated cheese, optional

Liver powder, optional

Grated apple, optional

1. Heat oven to 340°F/171°C. Line a baking sheet with parchment.

2. In the bowl of a food processor, combine all the ingredients. Pulse until mixed but still a bit chunky.

3. Press the dough evenly onto the prepared baking sheet. Alternatively, you can scoop the mixture into 40 portions for crunchier treats. Most dogs seem to like them crunchy.

4. Bake as a whole for 30–35 minutes, then cut into 40 portions while still warm. If baking individual treats, bake for about 9–11 minutes.

5. If you have a dog with no teeth, like my 5-pound rescue named Bisou, either bake them for a shorter time or crumble before serving.

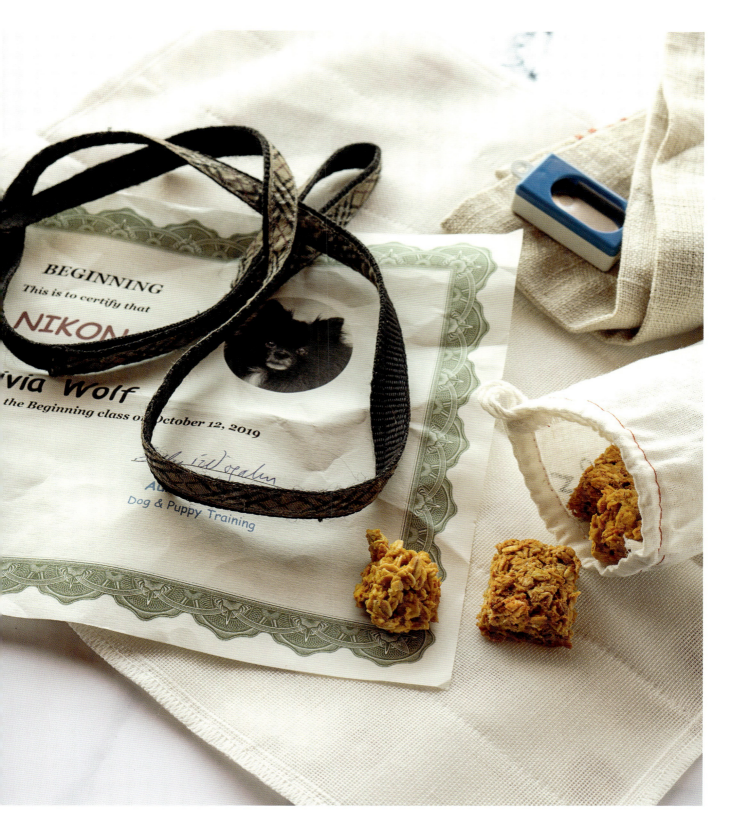

Acknowledgments

Thanks to my editor, Joe Davidson, and to our designer, Amanda Richmond, who were delightful from start to finish. They knew what they wanted and got us there. Bruce and I learned a lot. And speaking of Bruce, the photographer and my husband of thirty-something years, he takes a fine photo.

Writer Hannah Wallace was an invaluable resource with extensive knowledge of the subject matter. Hannah does a great interview, and her writing is informative without being wonky. And she is a pleasure to do business with. We had a couple of lovely lunches in her backyard, planning and eating and looking at hummingbirds.

Stylist Kyra Korbin added some beautiful pieces to our photos, and she has a good eye and totally got the look we wanted to achieve.

I want to thank the farms and shops that made us welcome throughout this project. Everybody is busy, and when we come in to photograph, it can be a bit disruptive. Did I say a bit? Well, a bit and a half. We were never rushed and never made to feel unwanted.

East Fork Cultivars hosted us for a couple of days and we were lucky enough to be able to get the full farm experience. It's hard to be a farmer! It made me glad we do edibles! The people at East Fork are great, and they make stellar craft hemp.

Noble Farms allowed us to shoot at their impressive indoor grow facility, after they suited us up in protective gear, of course. We photographed some of their beautiful buds and, of course, smoked them after. Great weed! Thanks, Will.

Golden Hour and Lumi Wellness both offer beautiful and calming environments; shooting there was a real treat. The dispensary, Jayne, is one of the loveliest in Portland, and they treated us like family.

Green Box is a Portland delivery service that offers a wide selection of the best pot in town, along with lots of cannabis products. Adrian, the owner, was able to hook me up with some terrific looking, and terrific smoking, flower, and he also helped me gain access to some top-of-the-line topicals and edibles. Thank you!

About 95 percent of the pottery in the book was crafted by ceramicist Odette Heideman from her studio, O. Atélier, in Maine. Custom pottery is a luxury I have never experienced before, and I treasure each piece for its elegant and rustic beauty.

The Jays and the Parkins allowed us to shoot in their beautiful homes, and I want that dreamy bathtub on page 37 for my birthday.

Research for the book required calling in products from around the country. We tried hundreds of different items and photographed the pieces we liked best. There are too many to list; they are all featured in the pages of this book, so you can see for yourself. I had the pleasure of getting a buzz (or two) from many of the pipes and vaporizers. The beauty and bath products featured were all excellent. Who knew? There is a whole world of new cannabis products that this book helped me to discover, and for that I'm grateful.

Our salespeople Keane, Mia, and Brandt were out and about and able to give me up to-the-minute info about new products on the market. Thanks for everything you three do.

A big thanks to the people who work in the kitchen and in packaging at Laurie + MaryJane. You are quite a delightful bunch.

To Claire and Ben for being patient models on the swing and in bed. To Ashley Dellinger, shown puffing in a chair at her perfectly curated CBD and wellness shop in Portland. And to the lovely Emily with flowers in her arms. Thank you all.

A ridiculous amount of thanks to Green Leaf Lab for their stellar work, it's been years now and they never disappoint. Kim, Eric, Julia, Briana, and Rowshan, we are indebted to you. We are kind of family now, and we feel so grateful.

Thanks to Titan's Kind, who make the super tasty candies featured on the Consuming and Acquiring page. We have shared a kitchen and we are grateful to Jonn, Andy, and the guys for their support, knowledge, and friendship.

Shout-out to "The Galley," and *Sensi* magazine for working with us as we transition to having Laurie + MaryJane produced in Santa Rosa, California.

And, finally, to friends and family who help keep us both sane and insane. Big thanks. For those of you who tried products, we appreciate it immensely.

Notes

Chapter 1: Cannabis: Past & Present

[1] Dave Olson, "Hemp Culture in Japan," *Journal of the International Hemp Association* 4, no. 1 (June 1997): 40–50.

[2] Jennifer Viegas, "World's Oldest Marijuana Stash Totally Busted," NBC News, December 3, 2008, http://www.nbcnews.com/id/28034925/ns/technology_and_science-science/t/worlds-oldest-marijuana-stash-totally-busted/#.XNn12NNKg_U.

[3] David Casarett, *Stoned: A Doctor's Case for Medical Marijuana* (New York: Current, 2015), 14–15.

[4] Ethan Russo et al., "Phytochemical and Genetic Analyses of Ancient Cannabis from Central Asia," *Journal of Experimental Botany* 59, no. 15 (November 2008): 4171–82.

[5] E. Joseph Brand and Zhongzhen Zhao, "Cannabis in Chinese Medicine: Are Some Traditional Indications Referenced in Ancient Literature Related to Cannabinoids?," *Frontiers in Pharmacology* 8 (March 2017): 108.

[6] Hampton Sides, "Science Seeks to Unlock Marijuana's Secrets," *National Geographic*, June 2015.

[7] Martin Booth, *Cannabis: A History* (New York: Picador, 2003), 73.

[8] W. B. O'Shaughnessy, "On the Preparations of the Indian Hemp, or Gunjah," *Provincial Medical Journal and Retrospect of the Medical Sciences* 5, no. 123 (February 1843): 363–69.

[9] "Marijuana Timeline," *Frontline*, https://www.pbs.org/wgbh/pages/frontline/shows/dope/etc/cron.html.

[10] "Did George Washington Grow Hemp?," George Washington's Mount Vernon, accessed on May 13, 2019, https://www.mountvernon.org/george-washington/facts/george-washington-grew-hemp.

[11] "Marijuana Timeline." (see #6)

[12] Advertisement in *Vanity Fair*, August 30, 1862, p. 134. Accessed on May 13, 2019, https://books.google.com/books?id=Kk4oAQAAMAAJ&dq=vanity+fair+1862&pg=RA1-PA134&hl=en#v=onepage&q=hasheesh&f=false.

[13] Stephen Siff, "The Illegalization of Marijuana: A Brief History," *Origins*, 7, no. 8 (May 2014).

[14] "Marijuana Timeline." (see #6)

[15] Siff, "The Illegalization of Marijuana."

[16] "Marijuana Timeline." (see #6)

[17] Siff, "The Illegalization of Marijuana."

[18] "Consequences of Marijuana Use & Policies: 70 Years Later, the Debate Continues," New York Academy of Medicine press release, April 30, 2014, https://www.nyam.org/news/article/consequences-of-marijuana-use-policies.

[19] Siff, "The Illegalization of Marijuana"; "Marijuana Timeline."

[20] "Marijuana Timeline."

[21] Siff, "The Illegalization of Marijuana."

[22] Wikipedia, s.v. "Controlled Substances Act," last modified December 1, 2019, 15:36, https://en.wikipedia.org/wiki/Controlled_Substances_Act.

[23] "Marijuana Timeline."

[24] John Walsh, "Q&A: Legal Marijuana in Colorado and Washington," The Brookings Institution, May 21, 2013, https://www.brookings.edu/research/qa-legal-marijuana-in-colorado-and-washington/.

[25] Justin Strekal at NORML, e-mail to author, May 6, 2019.

[26] See, for example, NORML's "Pennsylvania's Medical Marijuana Law" page at https://norml.org/legal/item/pennsylvania-medical-marijuana-law?category_id=835.

[27] See NORML's "About Marijuana" page at https://norml.org/aboutmarijuana.

28 Linda Carroll, "One in Seven U.S. Adults Used Marijuana in 2017," Reuters, August 27, 2018, https://www.reuters.com/article/us-health-marijuna-us-adults/one-in-seven-us-adults-used-marijuana-in-2017-idUSKCN1LC2B7.

29 "FDA-Approved Drug Epidiolex Placed in Schedule V of Controlled Substance Act," DEA press release, September 27, 2018, https://www.dea.gov/press-releases/2018/09/27/fda-approved-drug-epidiolex-placed-schedule-v-controlled-substance-act.

30 Craig Giammona, "Trendy Hemp Compound CBD Set for Big Boost from U.S. Farm Bill," *Bloomberg*, December 19, 2018, https://www.bloomberg.com/news/articles/2018-12-19/trendy-hemp-compound-cbd-set-for-big-boost-from-u-s-farm-bill.

31 CBD Certified class, Cultivation Classics, Portland, Oregon, May 17, 2019.

32 Ibid

33 Roger G. Pertwee, "Cannabinoid Pharmacology: The First 66 Years," *British Journal of Pharmacology* 147, Supplement 1 (January 2006): S163–S171.

Chapter 2: Cannabis Basics

1 J. Maroon and J. Bos, "Review of the Neurological Benefits of Phytocannabinoids," *Surgical Neurology International* 9 (April 2018): 91, doi:10.4103/sni.sni_45_18.

2 Noor Azuin Suliman et al., "Delta-9-Tetrahydrocannabinol (Δ9-THC) Induce Neurogenesis and Improve Cognitive Performances of Male Sprague Dawley Rats," *Neurotoxicity Research* 33, no. 2 (February 2018): 402–11, doi:10.1007/s12640-017-9806-x.

3 E. M. Rock et al., "Cannabinoid Regulation of Acute and Anticipatory Nausea," *Cannabis Cannabinoid Research* 1, no. 1 (April 1, 2016): 113–121, doi:10.1089/can.2016.0006.

4 X. Yu et al., "D-limonene Exhibits Antitumor Activity by Inducing Autophagy and Apoptosis in Lung Cancer," *OncoTargets and Therapy* 11 (April 4, 2018): 1833–1847, doi:10.2147/OTT.S155716.

Chapter 3: Cannabis as Medicine

[1] S. Ben-Shabat et al., "An Entourage Effect: Inactive Endogenous Fatty Acid Glycerol Esters Enhance 2-Arachidonoyl-Glycerol Cannabinoid Activity," *European Journal of Pharmacology* 353, no. 1 (July 1998): 23–31.

[2] Sunil K. Aggarwal, "Cannabinergic Pain Medicine: A Concise Clinical Primer and Survey of Randomized-Controlled Trial Results," *The Clinical Journal of Pain* 29, no. 2 (February 2013): 162–71.

[3] The National Academies of Sciences, Engineering, and Medicine, *The Health Effects of Cannabis and Cannabinoids: The Current State of Evidence and Recommendations for Research* (Washington DC: The National Academies Press, 2017).

[4] Christy Curran at Sam Brown Inc., public relations firm for Sativex, e-mail to author, June 21, 2019.

[5] The National Academies of Sciences, Engineering, and Medicine, *The Health Effects of Cannabis and Cannabinoids.*

[6] Ibid

[7] Michael Backes, *Cannabis Pharmacy: The Practical Guide to Medical Marijuana* (New York: Black Dog & Leventhal, 2017), 198.

[8] Ethan B. Russo, "Cannabis and Epilepsy: An Ancient Treatment Returns to the Fore," *Epilepsy & Behavior* 70, part B (May 2017): 292–97.

[9] D. Sulak, R. Saneto, and B. Goldstein, "The Current Status of Artisanal Cannabis for the Treatment of Epilepsy in the United States," *Epilepsy & Behavior* 70, part B (May 2017): 328–33.

[10] Scott Shannon et al., "Cannabidiol in Anxiety and Sleep: A Large Case Series," *The Permanente Journal* 23 (January 2019): 18–41.

[11] D. R. Blake et al., "Preliminary Assessment of the Efficacy, Tolerability and Safety of a Cannabis-Based Medicine (Sativex) in the Treatment of Pain Caused by Rheumatoid Arthritis," *Rheumatology* 45, no. 1 (January 2006): 50–52.

[12] Torsten Lowin, Matthias Schneider, and Georg Pongratz, "Joints for Joints:

Cannabinoids in the Treatment of Rheumatoid Arthritis," *Current Opinion in Rheumatology* 31, no. 3 (May 2019): 271–78.

[13] Balázs I. Tóth et al., "TRP Channels in the Skin," *British Journal of Pharmacology* 171, no. 10 (May 2014): 2568–81; Angelo A. Izzo et al., "Non-Psychotropic Plant Cannabinoids: New Therapeutic Opportunities from an Ancient Herb," *Trends in Pharmacological Sciences* 30, no. 10 (October 2009): 515–27.

[14] Antonio W. Zuardi et al., "Inverted U-Shaped Dose-Response Curve of the Anxiolytic Effect of Cannabidiol during Public Speaking in Real Life," *Frontiers in Pharmacology* 8 (May 2017): 259; M. M. Bergamaschi et al., "Cannabidiol Reduces the Anxiety Induced by Simulated Public Speaking in Treatment-Naïve Social Phobia Patients," *Neuropsychopharmacology* 36, no. 6 (May 2011): 1219–26; Antonio W. Zuardi et al., "Effects of Ipsapirone and Cannabidiol on Human Experimental Anxiety," *Journal of Psychopharmacology* 7, supplement 1 (January 1993): 82–88.

[15] A. W. Zuardi, F. S. Guimarães, and A. C. Moreira, "Effect of Cannabidiol on Plasma Prolactin, Growth Hormone and Cortisol in Human Volunteers," *Brazilian Journal of Medical and Biological Research* 26, no. 2 (February 1993): 213–17.

[16] E. M. Blessing et al., "Cannabidiol as a Potential Treatment for Anxiety Disorders," *Neurotherapeutics* 12, no. 4 (October 2015): 825–36.

[17] Scott Shannon et al., "Cannabidiol in Anxiety and Sleep: A Large Case Series," *The Permanente Journal* 23 (January 2019): 18–41.

Index

About the Authors

Laurie Wolf is a leader in the edibles community and an award-winning culinary entrepreneur. A graduate of the Culinary Institute of America, Laurie worked as a food stylist and editor before going on to pen four celebrated cannabis cookbooks and founding her own Portland-based edibles business, Laurie + MaryJane.

Mary Wolf is the daughter-in-law, co-author, and business partner of author Laurie Wolf. Their business Laurie + MaryJane has been providing high-quality, reliable edibles to the cannabis community since 2014.

Bruce Wolf was born in the Bronx and lived and worked as a photographer in Paris before moving to Portland, Oregon, with his wife, Laurie. In addition to collaborating with Laurie on a series of children's books and multiple cookbooks, Bruce continues to shoot commercially and has garnered numerous accolades for his work.

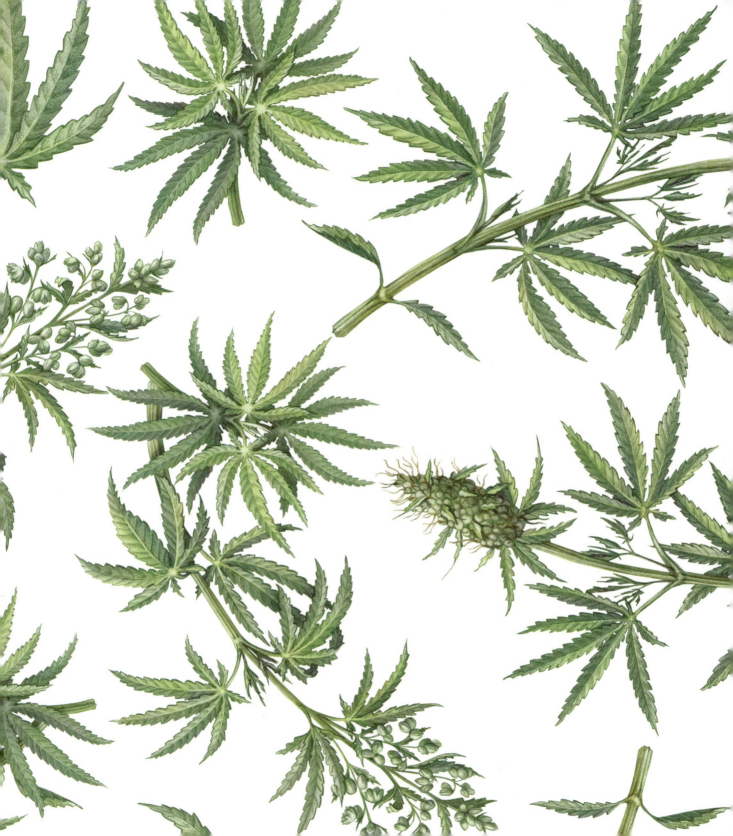

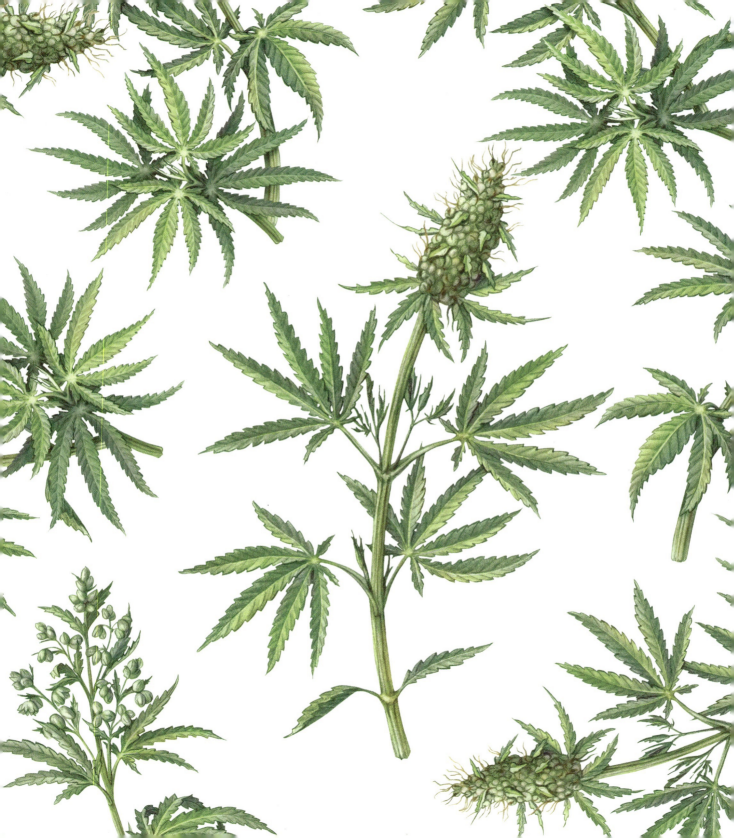